STOP DIETING & START LIVING

HOW TO PERMANENTLY LOSE YOUR UNWANTED WEIGHT, ELEVATE YOUR HEALTH & HAPPINESS. CHANGE THE WAY, YOU VIEW NUTRITION, FITNESS & DIETING!

WITHOUT STARVING...

Sakura Viotto

STOP DIETING & START LIVING

Abundant Press - Las Vegas, NV 89107 www.AbundantPress.com

Special discounts are available on quantity purchases by corporations, associations, and others. For details, contact the publisher. Orders by U.S. & International trade bookstores and wholesalers at: info@abundantpress.com. Printed in the United States of America- Library of Congress-in-Publication Data. Please note: If you find errors, like spelling or grammar, please send us an email.

Title: STOP Dieting & START Living
Sub-title: How to Permanently Lose Your Unwanted Weight, Elevate Your Health & Happiness. By Changing The Way, You View Nutrition, Fitness & Dieting! Without Starving.

Author: Sakura Viotto
1. The main category of the book — Health, Fitness, Wellness
First Edition: 2-28-2021 ISBN: 978-1-948287-29-6

The author has made every reasonable effort to be as accurate and complete as possible in the creation of this book and to ensure that the information provided is free from errors; however, the author/publisher/ reseller assumes no responsibility for errors, omissions, or contrary interpretation of the subject matter herein and does not warrant or represent at any time that the contents within are accurate due to the rapidly changing nature of the Internet.

Any perceived slights of specific persons, peoples, or organizations are unintentional.

Disclaimer

The information within this book is intended as reference material only and not as medical or professional advice. Information contained herein is intended to give you the tools to make informed decisions about your wellness, lifestyle, and physical and mental health. It should not be used as a substitute for any treatment that has been prescribed or recommended by your doctor. The information within this book must not be construed as a medical, therapeutic, or psychological treatment, nor are any such claims made.

Every reasonable effort has been made to ensure that the material within this book is true, correct, complete, and appropriate at the time of writing. Nevertheless, the authors do not accept responsibility for any omission or error, or for any injury, damage, loss, or financial consequences arising from the use of this material. The authors, promoters, and publishers are not healthcare professionals, and expressly disclaim any responsibility for any adverse effects occurring as a result of the use of the suggestions or information herein. This material is offered as practical, current information available about disease and health management for your own education and enjoyment.

If you suspect you have a disease of any kind, it is imperative that you seek medical attention. It is also recommended that you consult with a qualified healthcare professional before beginning any diet or exercise program. By accepting this information, you agree to hold Sakura Viotto & her associates, partners, and affiliates free of liability and damage, and you proceed on your own free will. You and you alone are solely responsible for the results that you produce. Do not continue unless you fully agree to these terms and conditions.

Important Note: It's important that you seek the advice and approval from your health care provider prior to making any drastic changes to your diet or exercise for any poor results you may attain when implementing the techniques or when following any guidelines set out for you in this book.

STOP DIETING & START LIVING

Table of Contents

The Problem with Diets of the Past
Chapter 1

It's a sad fact that most people reading this book right now are not on their first diet. Most probably aren't on their second, third, or even fourth diet, either. You're probably used to the merry go round of dieting, and each year, your weight creeps up higher and higher, and you're breaking the wrong sort of records.

It's not your fault unless you find out how to fix this problem and ignore the advice, choosing instead to get back on the same harmful, discouraging path you were on before.

What's wrong with the diets you've previously been on? A lot.

They Concentrated Heavily on Numbers

Most diets require you to have a strong background in math to understand and master them properly. From the calorie counting to the number of pounds, it's okay to lose in a week to the inches you gained in muscle and lost in fat – numbers swirling in your head can get overwhelming.

Some diets go even further than simple calories and have you performing math equations on every single meal you eat. Did you get the right number of carbs? Is the ratio of carbs to protein in the right vicinity?

What happens when you have to be a mathematician for each meal is that you get annoyed. You don't *feel* like counting and dividing and comparing and crunching numbers – so you just fly by the seat of your pants, do it all wrong, and wonder why you failed.

That or you get exhausted spending 10 minutes on math when you only have a 30-minute lunch break. Your diet *should* be focused on your wellbeing and how you're feeling, not on whether or not you got your math facts right.

They Focused on Extremes

Diets in your past probably went from one end of the spectrum to the other. Elimination diets where they have an all or nothing mentality aren't feasible – and they aren't enjoyable.

You need to learn how to eat for life, not for 30 days or six months. In some diets, you have to eliminate whole food groups – sometimes surviving solely on fattening meats and foregoing healthy fruits and vegetables.

Now, does that sound like a smart thing to do to your body? They're setting you up for failure because they're not doable for the long-term. If you look at a diet and start tallying up how many days, you'll "have to do it" to lose a certain number of pounds, then it's not a good diet to be on.

You Develop a Diet Mindset

A dieting mindset is crippling. If you become someone who is always thinking about dieting talking about dieting, and planning your life around dieting, then it's not leading a pleasant life.

Life should be about enjoying the time you spend with friends and family, about relishing the time you get to indulge in your favorite hobbies, about pursuing success and satisfaction in your career.

It shouldn't be an obsession with your body's faults and how you can take drastic measures to change the way you look. It should be about pursuing things that make you feel better – habits that deliver total wellness, including mental happiness – and a diet mindset isn't what that's about.

People with a diet mindset tend to do some of the following things:

- They frequently announce their diet progress to their friends and family – what they're planning to do, what they're doing, what they did, and where they failed.
- They don't realize it, but they often become critical of friends and family who aren't following the same regimen that they are – always verbally nitpicking on other people's actions to force them to change.
- They continually beat themselves up whenever they have slipups – always focusing on what they did wrong.

Instead of propping yourself up for yet another failure, and even more pounds packed onto your frame – make a commitment to change the way you diet starting this year.

A Better Way to Succeed with Dieting

Chapter 2

More than anything you just want to finally succeed. You're tired of failing and regaining even more weight than you had on you before. When New Year's Day rolls around, you're probably in a good state of mind.

You've motivated yourself for this day and you're ready to fight back against obesity. You start off great and probably thrive, watching the pounds fall off for days, weeks – maybe even months if you're one of the lucky few.

But it doesn't last. There comes a day when you're done. It starts with a few slip ups along the way. That turns into you beating yourself up for being a failure, and then one day you start to believe it – you accept defeat and quit until next New Year's Day (or maybe right before summer when you have to adopt your "bikini" mindset).

Forget About a Time Span

Are you looking to lose weight for a month – right before your 20th high school reunion? Or is this something you'd like to keep off for a lifetime? We both know the answer to this question, so why are you considering diets that aren't doable forever?

Lifelong habits are what you're after. So I want you to forget about how long you'll be dieting or how long it will take you to lose the weight you want to shed. I want you to just start today being a healthier person, period.

When you take the time pressure off of yourself, it opens you up to a whole new world of success. It won't feel comfortable, though. After all, every diet has promises of "2 pounds per week" or "She lost 15 pounds" with the small print of *results not typical that you like to ignore.

And what about those goals you have on your calendar? The ones like:

- Lose the last 15 pounds of baby weight by May 15th
- Lose 30 pounds before swimsuit season
- Lose 50 pounds before my high school reunion
- Lose 100 pounds before I walk down the aisle

What about those? You've put a ton of pressure on yourself with those goals. It's okay to have them – without an end date in mind. And it's great if you do reach those goals by the date you desired.

But what if you don't? If you don't, there's a tsunami of disappointment and failure labeling coming your way. There's an extreme diet fad in your near future as the deadline looms and you're not reaching your goal fast enough.

You end up doing more harm than good – and what really matters is that you become healthier, right? Once you analyze your body physically for its health needs (and yes, that may include weight loss), then you have to adopt a total mind and body wellness approach.

Use a Total Mind and Body Approach

Dieting isn't just about your body's size. It's about fueling your body for all of its needs and it's about working on your mindset so that you are all about self-care and not about wondering what others will think about you.

You need to approach dieting this New Year from head to toe, inside and out – on a physical and emotional level. This is going to be difficult for you to initially get used to, but once you do, you'll feel more powerful – and freer – than ever before.

You need to look at dietary changes that don't just help you get trim, but that help clear up your skin, help your heart function better, help you have more energy, help you get pregnant (if that's a goal), etc.

And you also need a diet that's not a diet in the traditional sense of the word. You want a way of eating. A way of feeding your body that makes it perform better for you. Something mindless that you can do without trying so hard.

Change the Word "Diet" to "Lifestyle"

The word *diet* can be a dirty word to some. It reminds them of being chained to a way of life that's limiting – something they dread. How about lifestyle from now on?

Instead of saying, "I can't eat that marbled steak – I'm on a diet and it has too many calories and too much fat," simply say, "Oh I like eating healthier, so I think I'll have lean chicken instead, but thanks!"

Instead of, "I have to burn 500 calories so I can have a Ho Ho today," say, "I'm going to take care of my body by giving it time to move today and increase its performance."

For more information about products that can support you on your Journey to Weight loss, & Amazing health visit:

SakuraNutraceuticals.com

Analyze Your Current Diet Mindset

Chapter 3

The first thing we have to do – before you ever put a single bite of "diet food" into your mouth and before you get up off the couch and get moving – it set your mind on the right path to success.

We have to take an honest account of where you are mentally. And it's kind of like how a doctor can look at stats going back 3 months – not just today's stats for your blood sugar levels.

You don't want to be all revved up and excited to lose weight today and trick yourself into a false sense of security that "you've got this." We have to get real and see where you've stood over the years.

Are You Going into This Expecting to Fail?

If you have failed before, you'll probably fail again, right? Not necessarily – but with an attitude like that, your chances increase. You have to go into this New Year lifestyle plan with expectations that you'll succeed.

Not wishful thinking – that's a very different concept. This has to be something where you "see" yourself trimmer, healthier, and more energetic than ever before based on what you plan to do.

If you get on a diet plan that's too restrictive, you can look at the odds and know right away that you're not going to stay on the plan 100% of the time. When you have a slip-up, you label it as such – and once you've done it, it doesn't matter if it's small – you've "failed."

This failure label gives you permission to go off the deep end. Instead of just eating a snack sized Snicker bar, you're suddenly on a death-by-chocolate bender.

There's a big difference between a 45-calorie snack and a 1,400-calorie dessert – and the effect it has on your body – but you won't care because you're being too rigid with yourself.

If the diet said no sweets and you broke the diet law, you should punish yourself. Get rid of your attitude that doesn't allow you to eat differently from time to time – and stop labeling things as "slip-ups" or "mistakes" as you plan your diet this New Year.

Another problem when you never expect success is that inevitably, you don't work as hard at the task as you would if you expected to succeed. You might not even be able to recognize that you're doing it, either.

If I told you right now that if you pushed yourself to work up your cardio this week and stuck to a reasonable diet plan and you'd lose every pound of weight that you wanted – 100% guaranteed, you'd do it.

But instead, you might be plotting your New Year diet in a way that just has you avoiding failure *for as long as you can* – so you might do cardio, but not nearly as hardcore as you would if you *knew* you'd succeed. You might eat okay, but not do it perfectly because failure is bound to happen anyway.

Have You Announced It to the World?

Traditionally, diet experts have advised people to set a goal and announce it to the world. They claimed that it made you accountable for your efforts. This should be a good thing, but it isn't.

There are several reasons why it's a better idea to quietly make this decision to lose weight on your own – and then keep it to yourself.

Announcing your weight loss goals *does* put pressure on yourself – and instead of having one person beating you up (yourself), you open the door to having everyone and their grandmother comment about what you're eating, and everything *they* believe you're doing wrong.

Studies also show that the simple task of announcing your goals satisfies you so much emotionally that it makes you work harder on the real things that matter – the actual nutrition and exercise portion of your diet plan.

It's as if announcing it was all you needed to do. But don't forget the guilt you feel – and shame – when, after announcing it to all of your friends, family, co-workers and Facebook friends, you have to then show them what a failure you've become when you don't achieve your wild 50 pounds in 5 weeks weight loss goals.

I know you want support – that's your real reason for announcing your goals to the world. You're hoping people will cheer you on and help you get past obstacles you encounter with your eating.

And yes, part of you might even appreciate (to a certain point), the nagging that occurs when you go to your Mom's house and try loading up on some fattening dessert, only to hear “tsk tsk” from a well-meaning loved one.

But remember that this journey you’re on toward better health isn’t about your friends and family – it’s about *you*. You’re the only one who needs to know this, and putting pressure on your acquaintances to babysit you isn’t fair to them, either.

When is it okay to let people know that you’re eating healthier or dieting? When they’re a source of the problem. If your grandmother bakes you 7 pies a week, it’s a problem. She needs to be told not to do that.

If your co-workers try pushing you into attending an endless stream of office celebrations with sweets, then you might say something in passing such as, “No thanks, I’m cutting down on my sugar intake.”

But you don’t need to make a declaration of your New Year diet plans, how much weight you plan to lose, and keep a running tally on Facebook for everyone to see of every meal you ate, each time you hit the gym, and how many calories you consumed in a 24-hour period.

There’s a lot of pressure to publicize your dieting, too. There are apps that will auto-Tweet your weight each week. There’s another app that tells everyone on social media when you skipped a workout at the gym.

You might as well walk around with a sign around your neck that tells everyone you meet that you need their approval to be happy because you’re inviting scorn, not just applause.

Do You Feel Guilt Associated with Diet Slip-Ups?

This is very common. In fact, if you're dieting and "slip up" in front of people without acknowledging your guilty feelings, people wouldn't even understand why!

Stop using words and phrases like "cheated" or "fell off the wagon." Your self-talk is the first thing you have to get under control so that you can stop *feeling* so negative about the choices you make.

This New Year, you should look at the long road ahead from this day to the rest of your life and realize that not every day has to be so regimented and restricted. Once you have the freedom to understand this concept, it makes it easier for you to have things that are outside your official diet plan without raking yourself over the coals for it.

That said, this doesn't mean your diet is now open so that you exist on nothing but donuts and brownies. But when you truly allow yourself to not feel food guilt anymore, you'll see how easy it is to indulge from time to time without turning it into an official (and unhealthy) binge.

Evaluate Your Existing Nutritional Intake

Chapter 4

Before you begin making nutritional changes, you have to see where you currently stand. Your goal is to identify both the habits you need to change and the habits you can feel good about keeping.

The Right and Wrong Way to Keep a Food Journal

Keeping a food journal requires two things: consistency and honesty. Without both of those, a food journal isn't going to help you replace bad habits with good ones!

You can keep a food journal on your PC, using a mobile app on your phone, or even using a traditional pen and paper approach. Some people even make video blog food journals and stick them on YouTube.

The goal is to record everything you eat and drink so that you can understand why you stall with weight loss if you reach a plateau or start gaining again. It's also supposed to keep you somewhat accountable in helping you stay on track with your diet plans.

Some people like to record everything as they eat every meal. You can record ingredients, portion sizes, caloric intake – down to the percentage of vitamins and other nutrients that the foods you eat offer.

But this can be too time consuming and daunting for many people. If your life is busy, it's okay to take a moment at the end of each day and record what you ate – as long as you don't forget about the time you went into the snack room and grabbed a croissant, or dipped into someone's candy jar on their desk.

You don't have to always keep a food diary, either. Some people like to do it forever, while others prefer to do it periodically just to help them see where their behavior is going wrong in a nutritional sense.

If you eat differently just because you're journaling, this can be a good or a bad thing. It's good if it helps you eat healthier and stick to your plan, but it's bad if the plan is so restrictive that you can't do it without monitoring yourself 24/7 like the food police.

You not only want to track your food, but the other elements that affect your nutrition. That includes where you ate – was it at the table or sitting on the couch mindlessly watching TV?

It also includes how you were feeling whenever you ate. Were you stressed and anxious (could that be why you just polished off a family sized bag of potato chips?) or were you content and eating mindlessly because you were in a comfortable mood and just wanted to feel relaxed and happy? Food diaries help pinpoint triggers for you.

Some people find that it helps to write down their food goals for the day at the beginning of each food journal entry. For example, you can jot down how many servings of grains or fruit you want to try to get into your diet.

You can even cross them off as you consume them, so that you're looking at what you *do* eat, rather than what you *can't* have. A food journal can help you figure out which foods you need help getting more of or getting less of.

A food journal won't do any good unless you go back later and actually read it. Look at your weight loss and other health factors for the week and then look back to see where the foods you ate helped or hurt the efforts.

What Are Your Portions Like?

Portions in America have gotten out of control when it comes to restaurant meals – we already knew this. But it's the same in our own homes. We put way more on our plate than we really need to fuel our bodies.

Portion recommendations differ according to your age, your weight, your gender, and whether or not you're pregnant or breastfeeding. But you still need to know a starting point to see where you currently are with portions.

It might help to go ahead and fix your plate and then measure the foods so that you can see what you've been doing. Don't measure before putting them on your plate because that doesn't tell you what you've been used to doing.

You might think you've only been eating a half a cup of mashed potatoes, but get shocked when you measure and realize it's actually been 2 ½ cups this whole time.

Do you fill your entire plate – and if so, is it a large dinner plate? Plate sizes have grown with portion sizes in America, to help fool us into thinking we're eating a normal amount.

What about *how* you fill your plate? Have you noticed that the biggest portions on your plate are the meats or fats, with the grains or vegetables being the tiniest portions?

It's important to see how your plate stacks up now against the future health and wellness plate you plan to prepare in the New Year on whatever diet plan you choose to follow.

Are You a Grazer or a Fueler?

Some people snack all day long – from the time they wake up and pour their first cup of coffee to the moment they slip into bed with a little before-slumber snack. This is known as a grazer.

Grazers don't usually sit down to three square meals a day – breakfast, lunch, and dinner. Instead, they keep their bodies going all day long by snacking. The key is in knowing *why* you're snacking.

Strategically, this can be a helpful dietary plan – like those who eat 6 small meals a day rather than three large ones. But if you're snacking because you're stress eating, or snacking on the wrong kinds of food all day (like propping your body up with a non-stop sugar rush), then it becomes a problem.

Fuelers are different types of eaters. They fuel up with a hearty breakfast, work all morning, and stop for more nutritional fuel at lunch – doing the same at dinnertime until the day is done.

They choose *not* to snack in between meals. Some people prefer this because they like how it feels to eat and fill up rather than never get that specific "full" feeling that grazing lacks.

Either way, you can lose weight and feel great. The key is in choosing healthy foods that keep hunger pangs at bay, but which don't stuff you like a Thanksgiving turkey each meal.

It might be easier for you to transition from foods that aren't as nutritionally sound to foods that offer a multitude of health benefits if you keep eating on the same schedule that you always have – at least for the time being.

You might want to switch schedules after a while if you decide to, once you're familiar with the new foods and feeling confident that you enjoy the meal plans you're working with.

For more information about products that can support you on your Journey to Weight loss, & Amazing health visit:

SakuraNutraceuticals.com

What Kind of Movement Is Your Body Getting?

Chapter 5

Some people think they're more active than they really are. Along with diet, your body needs to move to maximize the benefits of your eating plan and help you get as healthy as possible.

Let's take a look at three different types of lifestyles so that you can see where you currently are – because you might be on a higher level of activity than you realize and therefore need more calories to sustain your body's energy throughout the day.

Extreme Sedentary Lifestyles

It takes a lot to be sedentary. Most people aren't sedentary at all – they're somewhat active, going to their jobs, grocery shopping, attending their kids' sporting events or participating in family activities.

Sedentary people are known to have what's called sitting disease. That's all they do – sit. They *might* get up to go to the restroom, their bed, or the kitchen – but other than that, they're couch potatoes the rest of the time.

Now being *home* doesn't necessarily mean you're sedentary – even if you happen to sit quite a bit. If you're active around the house during the day off and on, then you get bumped up to the moderate movement category.

Try to keep a little log of the hours you spend sitting down – even if it's at a desk working in an office or from home – compared to the times when you're up moving around.

You can track a week or so, but make sure it's an average week for you – not one when you happen to have a lot going on that requires more movement than usual.

Write down what it is you like to do during your sedentary moments, too. Is it sitting and staring out the window? Reading a good book? Playing video games? Watching a good TV show or movie?

Your goal later will be to incorporate some of your favorite activities into more physical movement. For example, there are video game consoles like Kinect that require movement so you're not being sedentary at all.

Moderate Movement

The moderate movement level has a different meaning. It's all about light activity – more than sedentary, but not quite hardcore exerciser. The moderate mover doesn't always work to include exercise into their daily routine, but they happen to get physical activity throughout their day.

Or, it's possible that they lead sedentary lifestyles but *do* work in a small amount of exercise in their day, such as a 30-minute walk around the neighborhood after dinner.

People who fall under this category could be students in college who walk from class to class and across campus, people who work in an office setting who are constantly getting up and down out of their chairs, or workers who have jobs where they're continually moving like doctors or blue-collar laborers.

When you start tracking your movement, look to see if you have 120-180 minutes of movement each week.

If so, even if you're not working up a complete sweat during this time, then you fall under the moderate movement category.

Exercise Elite

The exercise elite are those who are extremely active. These people don't just get more movement throughout their day due to basic decisions like walking to deliver a message instead of emailing – they actually do that *and* work in an abundance of exercise that gets their hearts beating before each day is done.

The elite exercisers are those who are considered athletes. Do you regularly play a sport or participate in athletic events like marathons that you train for continually? If so, you're an active person – not moderately active or sedentary.

Some careers require you to be highly physically active. This would include a soldier, some agriculture laborers, or other industry workers. If you get anywhere from six to 10 hours a week or more is considered extremely active.

Make a record, like you do of your nutritional intake, of how much movement you get. Not necessarily formal exercise – because all movement is good for you – but times when you're up off the couch, putting your legs and arms in motion.

Tally up the hours to see if you qualify for moderate or extreme exercise levels and then you can choose a meal plan that helps you fuel your body. The last thing you want is to cut calories to such a deficit that you weaken your energy stores and become *less* active and less able to lose weight effectively.

What Other Health Needs Should Your Diet Assist?

Chapter 6

There are plenty of diets to choose from, but only certain ones will help you get other health problems under control. Diets that target specific health conditions or diseases can make it easier on your body to lose the weight because the diet is focused on whole body health.

By selecting a diet that treats the whole body, you're more likely to have long term success because you'll be getting and feeling healthier as you lose weight. The focus of a diet that shows you how to eat well and get fit will be on improving your lifestyle rather than as a quick fix.

Heart Disease

A lot of people struggle with health issues that can cause heart disease. One of the symptoms of this health issue early on can be high blood pressure readings. So if you have a problem keeping your blood pressure under good control, you'll want to look for a diet that can help you with that.

One of those diets is the DASH diet. This is an acronym for Dietary Approach to Stop Hypertension and it's one of the diets that the National Institutes of Health recommends for people who have hypertension.

You can either use the regular DASH eating plan or the one that's geared toward lowered sodium meals.

There are no special foods to buy - you simply eat healthy ones like fruits and vegetables, low fat dairy and lean meats.

If the DASH plan isn't what you wanted, there are other diet plans beneficial to heart disease reversal and prevention. Other diets beneficial for the heart are the TLC diet, the Ornish diet, Flexitarian diets, a vegan or vegetarian diet, and many more.

Diabetes

The DASH diet also helps people with diabetes. Another health issue you want to look at when you're searching for the right diet plan for you is your glucose control.

If you've been diagnosed with pre-diabetes or diabetes, you want that stabilized to either prevent getting full blown diabetes or getting it under control to stave off long term health effects that diabetes can sometimes cause.

You can use the DASH diet for treating diabetes as well, but another healthy diet for treating this condition is the Weight Watchers program. Weight Watchers puts an emphasis on making healthy food choices, though you're allowed to eat whatever you like.

The plan will give you well rounded meals that include healthy foods and will give you the guidelines to help you with the portion sizes as well. This plan also focuses on something that impacts diabetes - and that's exercise.

By choosing a diet plan that promotes exercising, you can bring your diabetes under control and have A1c levels within recommended ranges.

If you don't want to try the DASH diet, there are others – including the Biggest Loser diet, the Engine 2 diet, the Mayo Clinic diet, the Glycemic Index diet and more.

Anti-Aging

The foods that you eat can take a toll on your organs. If you eat a diet that's high in fat and red meats, not only does it show up on your skin, but it can cause cellular aging within the body, too.

Diets that can help with anti-aging have one thing in common. The diet is centered on foods that are natural and will result in a safe rate of weight loss. The foods in any anti-aging diet will include whole grains because fiber helps your blood vessels stay in good shape.

A diet that's rich with anti-aging properties will also have fish and lean meats as the protein suggestions for your meals. Fish is rich in Omega-3 and can also assist users with maintaining cognitive skills including fighting against memory loss.

The anti-aging diet will also have you eating plenty of antioxidant bearing fruits and vegetables. Not only do you get the benefit of eating foods that help in the fight against cancer, but these foods help your eyes fight against conditions that would attack your eyesight.

Cancer Prevention

It used to be that cases of cancer were less common than they are today. Some of the reasoning behind that is because we have better early detection tests, but some of it is because more and more people rely on a diet that's loaded with foods that don't give their bodies the benefits of cancer fighting foods.

It's easy to fall into the habit of grabbing whatever is fast and convenient. But eating healthier really doesn't take any more time - it simply takes commitment and planning ahead.

The long-term benefits to your body are well worth that. Look for diets that will help your body give you a boost up on cancer prevention. The American Journal of Clinical Nutrition published a story that showed the benefits of one diet against the risk of getting breast cancer.

That was the Mediterranean diet. In this diet, users avoid the saturated fats and processed foods that contain ingredients that aren't good for the body. Instead, people who follow the Mediterranean diet can help keep cancer at bay by eating foods rich in antioxidants and fish containing Omega 3.

If you're looking for a diet that will give you long term benefits, this is a good one - especially if you have a family history of certain cancers.

Inflammation

Some people struggle with inflammation. Whether it's short or long term, inflammation in the body can make you feel miserable. You want to have an eating plan that will give your body relief from inflammation.

Diets that contain sugary foods or foods that are high in saturated fats can trigger certain inflammation. If you've been struggling with any kind of inflammatory disease or you have arthritis in your joints that seems to get worse, what you're eating could be what's triggering your flare ups.

Diets that help treat inflammations are diets that suggest avoiding white foods like sugar and white flour. Vegetarian diets are good diets for people who have inflammation.

Even eating a vegetarian meal plan a few times a week can make a difference in how you feel. Select foods like whole grains, baked fish, dark leafy greens, almonds, low-fat dairy, tomatoes and beets.

All of those foods are good as part of a balanced meal to help you lose weight, but you'll notice that you feel better when you eat foods that target inflammation. One of the diets that you might want to check out if you're struggling with inflammation or arthritis is the Paleo diet.

Energy

If you seem to struggle with not having enough energy to get through the day, you'll want to look for a diet that can help to boost your energy levels. The kinds of diets that can help you to get your stamina back are diets that are loaded with high fiber foods and foods that help keep your energy level up during your waking hours.

If you're looking to boost your energy, then you need to be careful around low carb diets because carbs give you energy and the more complex the carb, the higher amount of energy it gives you as it turns the carb into fuel for your body.

If energy is a side health issue for you, then you might benefit from a diet plan that requires multiple small meals throughout the day. That helps keep your metabolism boosted so that you can function better.

Infertility

Carrying too much extra weight can make it more difficult to conceive. If you need to lose weight and you're struggling with infertility, there are diets that can help you with that health issue.

Certain foods affect your hormonal levels and can help you with ovulation. The nutrients in some foods play a role in your reproductive ability and your hormones need these nutrients in order for you to conceive.

You want a diet that's rich in green, red and yellow vegetables and you want to choose organic foods whenever possible. Eat a lot of fish and stay away from processed foods.

Get your servings of fiber because that helps your hormones get the balance that they need. A good example of a diet for infertility would be the Mediterranean diet.

Other Health Concerns

Sometimes habits we have can really do a number on our health. But there are diets that can help us stop continuing with bad habits. Smoking can be curbed through a diet and the foods in a healthy diet can help repair damage done to the body from smoking.

To stop smoking, look for a diet that offers up plenty of hard, crunchy food. Some foods that aren't good for you actually make smoking taste better while other foods, such as apples, make a cigarette taste worse.

Stress is another health issue that some dieters deal with. There are diets that can help you fight stress.

These diets suggest stress fighting foods such as oatmeal, complex carbs, fruits and vegetables.

For those with allergies, eating right while dieting can sometimes be challenging. There's some truth to the saying that an apple a day keeps the doctor away. Apples are good in diets for allergies and so are red grapes. Nuts, onions and garlic can also fight allergies. Look for a diet that includes these helpful foods.

Indigestion is never fun. Normally, a diet that suggests lots of fruits and vegetables is beneficial for all users - but not for people with indigestion. If you suffer from this, you'll want to stay away from diets that are filled with acidic foods, which worsen indigestion.

Avoid citric and tomato-based foods as well as coffee, garlic and spicy foods. Sometimes, you'll only need to cut them out in the evening hours, but you can enjoy them early on in the day.

If you want to leave insomnia behind, you can do it naturally through diet. There are foods that contain tryptophan, which helps you sleep. Diets high in whole grain foods, fruits and vegetables and low-fat dairy products can help you stop tossing and turning.

If you want a diet that helps you heal from skin problems, diets that are heavy in fish, especially salmon, can help. Blueberries are great at correcting skin problems, too.

You want to avoid pineapples because they can cause flare-ups and so can certainly spices. So, diets that focus on spices as a way of preparing meals wouldn't be good for you.

Did you know that certain foods can actually trigger a headache? They can - because some foods contain tyramine and can bring on a headache. Foods containing tyramine are processed meats, beans, soups, nuts and many cheeses.

For people who deal with headaches, avoiding these foods can stop the cycle. With the exception of eating beans, a vegetarian diet can help eliminate headaches.

You never want to choose a diet plan solely based on how many pounds it can help you whittle off your body in the shortest amount of time. Instead, you want to look good *and* feel great!

You want longevity and good health with your new, trim figure. So, it's important that you base your diet plan choice for the New Year on its health-benefiting traits according to what you need for your body.

Do You Want to Officially Diet or Get Healthy?

Chapter 7

Your first instinct is to jump on a diet plan that will crank up your metabolism and help you burn more calories than you take in so that the weight falls off. But you want the all over body and mind health benefits.

Choosing a Diet Plan That Works for You

Consider your health issues first. If you have high blood pressure and your doctor is telling you that he or she is concerned, then maybe a Weight Watcher's diet where you can eat anything as long as you control a certain number of points isn't right for you.

You need to be realistic with your health because it doesn't matter how skinny you get if you end up hospitalized due to side health factors you chose to ignore in the name of fitting into a smaller size.

Look at what's required of your schedule. If you are a completely busy person, then it might be wise for you to choose a diet that might include foods that are either pre-packaged or easy to prepare ahead of time.

If your schedule is packed, it might not be feasible for you to sit there constantly measuring and analyzing each bite you put in your mouth.

On the other hand, if you work from home and have a little more time to utilize, then you might want to choose a meal plan where you *can* take advantage of those perks by preparing fresh foods for all of your daily meals.

Pick a diet that allows your favorite foods. If you're lucky enough to not be suffering from any additional health issues, then you might want to choose a diet that lets you consume some of your favorite foods.

For example, if you're a big meat eater, it would be cruel of you to restrict your entire diet to a vegan or vegetarian diet seven days a week. Going meatless a few times makes sense for future health reasons, but there's no reason to jump to extremes that will only make you miserable.

If budget is a concern, look for a diet that suits yours. You might really love the idea of Jenny Craig's diet plan, but finding out that the weekly meals cost as much as they do could shoot a hole in those plans.

Don't let it become an excuse for you to eat unhealthily, though. Some people complain that fruits and vegetables are too costly, but there are plenty of options that are affordable.

You can cut down on costs by not buying organic produce, by buying whole pieces instead of those that are prepackaged and already cut up and pre-washed for you, and by shopping for items that are in season.

Make Small Changes That Improve Health

Use special nutrition-friendly plates. You can buy smaller plates – and even plates that have the right portion control on them, like a space for fruits, a space for grains, a space for vegetables, and a space for protein.

Resist the urge to add salt and sugar. Your foods are already packed with plenty of salt and sugar, yet we tend to add much more because our taste buds have grown used to it.

You have to wean yourself off of extra salt and sugar. As you go through withdrawals and allow your taste buds to get back to a normal state, you'll realize that you need less and less sugar and salt – and you can taste them naturally in the foods that you buy.

Learn how to pair carbs and proteins. Carbs are good – they give you energy that you need to refuel and keep going throughout the day. But eaten by themselves, and your energy spikes and then crashes.

Instead, you should learn how to pair a carb with a filling protein that keeps you feeling satisfied for a longer period of time. For example, let's say you want some sort of bread breakfast like toast.

That's okay – but eat it with a piece of string cheese or some yogurt so that the protein works to stabilize your blood sugar and keep you from feeling hungry faster.

Don't skip meals – or *should* you? For a long time, the advice was that you never skip a meal – especially breakfast. It was touted as a way to rev up your metabolism and help you lose weight.

But now experts disagree. Some say that if you're not hungry – don't eat! You have to make this decision yourself based on your habits. Do you tend to skip a meal and then binge when you finally *do* sit down to eat? If so, then it might be a good idea to stick to traditional thinking.

Focus on what you can *add to* your diet, not what you have to lose. For example, try to get a rainbow of fruits and vegetables into your diet each day. Think of how you can work it into your meal plan, like this:

- Breakfast: Orange cantaloupe
- Mid-Morning Snack: Handful of blueberries
- Lunch: Raw or steamed broccoli
- Afternoon Snack: Red strawberries
- Dinner: Yellow squash

If you can work in more, do it! Try to make a list of a variety of colorful foods that you like in both the fruits and vegetable categories. Test things you haven't even tried yet, too.

Natural Ways to Burn More Calories Throughout Your Day
Chapter 8

There are many ways you can go from sedentary to moderate or even elite exercise enthusiast. You can join classes for fitness, invest in exercise equipment, and commit to regimented programs that get your moving more.

But this year, you should also be working toward increasing your average, everyday activities – because it's in this area that the efforts can truly add up and amount to better health.

Use a Pedometer

If you don't have time to get your fitness routine done every day, there's still a way that you can burn calories. There's a simple and inexpensive device you can get that can help you to knock off calories and pounds.

You can get a pedometer. Studies have shown that using a pedometer helps people on their weight loss journey because it gives them a way to see their efforts. They get to see progress daily.

By walking 10,000 steps in a day, you'll walk about 5 miles. When you have a pedometer along with a healthy diet plan, you'll lose weight steadily. The best thing about a pedometer is that you can get in your daily steps even while you're just going about your regular routine. You'll find that you're looking for ways to add to your step count - such as parking further away from the door of the store when you have to go shopping.

You can start slow if you're not used to doing anything physical and you can increase your progress a little bit each day until you're at the point where you're meeting or exceeding your daily step goal.

Experience Short Bursts of Exercise at Work

Another way that you can burn more calories can be done while you're at work. Even if you have a job that requires you to sit at a desk for most of the day, you can still get in some quick and effective moves that will help you stay fit.

You can do seated leg lifts right in your office chair. Simply lift your left leg and hold it out straight. Count to ten and then lower the leg slowly. Switch to the right leg and do the same. Alternate each leg for a few minutes to tighten those muscles.

If you have an area at work where you can be alone for a few minutes, you can knock out some pushups using either the floor or against the wall. Sit ups are good, too if you can find some space to do them in.

While you're standing at the water machine or waiting for someone at the office, you can do standing leg lifts. Stand on one leg and bend the other one at the knee so that you're raising the heel of your foot toward your rear end. Hold until the count of ten then slowly put your foot down. Repeat with the other leg.

Walking during work is a great way to exercise and you can take a brisk walk around your office area. You can also go for lunch walks. If you don't have the time to get outside at your office, walk your office building to deliver messages instead of using email. Skip using the elevator and instead, choose to use the stairs. Each time you use the stairs, those steps add up. Get rid of your desk chair and instead, sit on a large exercise ball. Using an exercising ball helps you strengthen your abdominal muscles while you're exercising. You're also exercising your calf muscles at the same time.

You can do toe raises while you're at a desk. With the heel of your foot on the ground, lift the toes of your foot upward and hold for the count of ten. Lower your foot and switch to the other foot.

You can burn calories and get your rear in shape at the same time by squeezing your glutes. You can do this while you're waiting to go into a meeting or even get in a few quick squeezes while in the restroom.

Jumping jacks are another easy exercise that you can do at the office. You can also run-in place or do walking lunges for a couple of minutes at a time several times throughout the day. A couple of minutes here and there to do these simple exercises can easily add up to a workout.

Make Cleaning a Physical Activity

Sometimes, there's just not time to get to the gym or to go for a walk because life can get busy - or maybe you'd rather do anything else than commit to a daily exercise routine. You don't want to lose the momentum you have going and there are other ways you can shed calories.

One often overlooked way of burning calories besides heading for the gym is cleaning. Whenever your body is in motion, it's burning calories. If you don't have time to exercise or you hate to exercise, then start cleaning!

The more vigorous the cleaning, the more calories you'll burn. Just sweeping the kitchen floor can burn 112 calories. If you have carpet in your home, that can be a good thing to help you burn calories because every time you vacuum, you can knock off 119 calories.

Dusting the knickknacks or the furniture can net you a burn of 85 calories. Making a bed burns 68 calories. If all you did was work for half an hour and you made your bed, dusted the room and vacuumed, you'd burn a total of 272 calories.

If it took you an hour, you'd double that number. Before you clean your bedroom, if you decide to do some laundry first, you'll burn 36.5 in calories for every 15 minutes you spend doing laundry.

When it's time to clean your floors, think about the calories you'll burn while you're getting your home in great shape. Every time you scrub the floors, you burn 258 calories for every hour.

Spring cleaning your house burns more calories and can give you the same vigorous workout you'd get if you were going hard at it on a treadmill. Doing simple chores burns calories, too - and if you hand wash the dishes instead of putting them in the dishwasher, you'll take off 78 calories. Chores where you have to work up a sweat can really take off the calories. If you need to clean your bathroom, you'll burn 200 calories and that's every half hour you devote to it.

If you live in a home that has more than one bathroom, you get to multiply that loss by the number of bathrooms you have for every half hour that you clean.

The best part about knocking off calories through cleaning your house, besides having a clean house at the end of all the chores is that it doesn't all have to be done all at once like working out at the gym does.

Instead of spending hours cleaning, you can clean in short bursts for 10-15 minutes at time throughout the day and still get the same benefit you would if you'd worked straight through.

Do Some Outside Work to Burn More Calories?

Besides cleaning inside the house, doing work outside is great for getting rid of calories, too. You can take your dog for a walk around your neighborhood and depending on your weight, you can easily burn 150 calories or more for every half hour you spend walking your pet.

The things you do to make the outside of your house look nice can be a good way for you to exercise as well. Washing the outside windows of your home knocks off 102 calories in a thirty-minute time span and will help make your house sparkle!

Mowing the yard is an outside activity that will burn calories fast. If you're 200 or more pounds overweight, you can burn over 276 calories for each half an hour it takes you to mow. So, if you mow for an hour, you'll burn over 550 calories.

Washing your car can burn up to 204 or more calories every hour. If you like flower gardening, you can have a yard filled with pretty flowers and take off 272 calories for every hour you spend giving your home some curb appeal.

Engage in Fun Activities to Better Your Health

Burning calories doesn't all have to be chore related. Don't forget that fun activities that help you relax can also burn calories. Dancing is one of those activities. You can dance at home, with friends or in an organized group class.

However, you do it, you'll be twisting and turning those calories right off. Dancing can burn 240 or more calories per half hour depending on the type of dancing that's involved. The more complex and the faster the pacing, the more calories you'll burn.

Many people enjoy roller-skating - but you might not know that roller-skating can easily burn 350 or more calories for every half an hour that you spend doing it. For people who like to engage in activities like kickboxing, they can burn over 480 calories every half hour they spend doing it.

If you take a kickboxing class, in one hour, you could burn 960 calories - and not only are you getting fit, but you could also be learning some helpful self-defense moves while you're at it.

Playing racquet type games such as tennis, badminton or squash can burn a lot of calories in a short amount of time. Because it's faster paced, squash burns the most, coming in at 533 calories for every half an hour spent in a game.

Tennis burns almost 400 and badminton 285. If you like to go bowling, you can take off 308 calories for every hour you spend doing it. Golf is a sport where you may not be going fast, but you can walk up to five miles if you play one round of 18 holes!

There are some days when you don't feel like doing anything outside or inside the house, even if it is fun. On days like that, if you spend half an hour playing with your children or with your pets, you can still burn calories. Playing with your children will burn 241 calories and playing with pets will burn the same amount.

Check-In Milestones Throughout the Year
Chapter 9

This year, it's important to step away from your daily check-in habit because you're turning this into a lifetime change, not an obsession. There are monthly, quarterly and semiannual or annual logs you can keep to ensure you're on the right track.

When you're on a quest to lose weight and get your body in shape for a healthier you, you want to have some milestones in place. Sometimes in enthusiasm for starting a new health journey, we can get our nutrition out of balance or we can do too much of a good thing.

Monthly Makeovers

Monthly makeovers are something that you want to schedule the time for. There are certain things you want to keep an eye on throughout the month. One of those things is your nutrition.

Sometimes you can go by the way you feel. If you start to feel tired and run down, then you might not be getting all of the nutrients you need. Check what you've been eating to make sure that you're covering all the right food groups.

If you see an area that you've been a little lax with, then you can alter your diet to get where you need to be. If you can't figure out what's lacking in your nutrition, you can get your doctor to do a simple blood test to tell you what you should add to your diet.

Remember that too much of a vitamin or mineral can potentially also have negative effects - just as too little can. That's why it's important that you check what you've been eating.

You can also tell if you're getting enough nutrients in the foods you eat by how fast you're losing weight. If you start to lose weight too fast that's a sign that you're not replacing the fuel that your body is burning.

Healthy eating always goes hand in hand with its partner - exercise. If you're not exercising enough, sometimes that will show up as a weight loss plateau. You'll just stop losing weight.

So, if that's the case, you'll need to step up the output a bit. A regular exercise routine helps you lose the weight, but it also helps tone areas of your body that need toning – plus it keeps your organs healthy.

But just as what you eat is important, how much you exercise is important, too. You don't want to push your body to the extent that you're straining and spraining things in your body.

Too much exercise will cause you to lose too much weight and will send your body into a starvation mode. When that happens, your body will slow the metabolism down as part of its safety mechanism. You don't want that to happen because then a slower metabolism makes it more difficult to lose weight.

Stepping onto the scale during regular weigh ins can help show you if you're making progress in the direction you want to take.

You should make sure that your weight is coming off at healthy levels - and that's at the 1-2 pounds a week that doctors recommend.

Any faster than that after the initial first week and it's too fast. When you weigh yourself, you can see how you've progressed and whether or not you need to do more to continue losing.

You shouldn't be so focused on the numbers on your scale that you get down emotional if you notice your weight stayed the same from the last weigh in or if you've gained since then.

Your weight will fluctuate according to several factors, so if you get one weigh in that isn't what you want, just stay on the path. It will change. The number on the scale isn't always the best indicator of true weight loss.

You want to pay attention to your body's measurements every month. Measure your chest area, your waist and hips to see if those numbers are going down. That – plus how your clothes fit - are usually a better indicator of weight loss than the scale.

Quarterly Milestones

As well as monthly makeovers for your weight, you also want to look at how you're doing quarterly. During the first period of a new weight loss and fitness journey, toward the end of the first quarter is when enthusiasm starts to lag.

Sometimes this can be due to being in the same exercise routine for too long. That's why it's important that you not stick with the same exercise routine. Not only can boredom be a problem, but not changing anything in your diet or exercise is what causes your weight to become stagnant.

You have to shake things up and the best time to do that is about every three months or so. Maybe the time of year has you stuck inside now and you can't get out in the fresh air and go for a run the way that you used to.

Find another set of exercises that you enjoy to take the place of running during those months. Now might be a great time to sign up for a vigorous dance class or to take some martial arts classes to shake your body up.

If you're used to exercising alone and you feel the need to make some changes in your routine and you're looking for some accountability and motivation, consider getting an exercise partner or personal trainer.

You also want to check to see what it is that your body is saying to you. Check out how your skin is looking and how your hair looks. Your diet and exercise routine should not make your skin look dry or your hair lackluster.

You shouldn't be stuck dealing with the same problem area of your body and not have noticed any changes in it by now. Sometimes you have to adjust your nutrition and physical activity to find what works for you.

In the first quarter, your body should have changed in some way. You should notice that there are inches gone from that area or that it's firmer than it was before. You also want to look at your BMI numbers to see what they are. By now, there should be a change in your BMI - even if it's not a very big change yet.

Take a look at your weight loss goals and see if you are where you wanted to be since you started your journey.

Seeing progress, even in small increments, can help you stick with it for the long haul.

Remember that it's okay to make changes. What worked for you in the beginning may not work for you now. It's okay to change your diet, your routine - *and* your goals. The object is for you to get healthy and that's what matters.

Semi Annual or Annual Check-Ups

Getting a semi-annual or an annual check-up is very important when you're on a weight loss, get fit life change. Seeing changes on the outside doesn't always indicate that what's going on within your body is what needs to be happening.

The only way that you can tell if everything is well inside is to get tests done at your doctor's office. He or she can run a blood panel and test to see that all of your numbers are at a good (or improving) level.

You want to get your glucose level tested. You'll want an immediate one that will tell you what it is at the time, but you'll also want an A1c - because this will tell you if your glucose levels were within range for the previous three months.

Get your cholesterol tested as well. High cholesterol should go down with the right diet. You want to make sure that you're eating the right diet that's targeting any of the health problems that you have.

Because it can be easy to get off track with the vitamin levels you need when you're dieting, it's important to ensure that your body is getting all that it needs of each vitamin and mineral.

So, get your vitamin levels checked. You'll also need your blood pressure tested, which is usually customary at any doctor's visit. With diet and exercise, your blood pressure should be within the normal range.

By getting the blood panel done and having your blood pressure checked, you'll see how you've been faring. If your numbers come back and they're not within the acceptable range, that's an indicator that something isn't working.

If you know that you've been exercising faithfully, then a clue would be that your diet isn't working. Even if you've seen weight loss with the diet, that doesn't mean that it's targeting your health problems. You want the diet that *does*.

So, if you've been on one diet for six months and you've lost inches but your glucose levels are still out of control, then it's time to switch to another diet. Sometimes, even if a diet is outlined to help with one health issue such as the DASH diet does with hypertension, it doesn't work for certain people.

The reason is that our bodies are all different and what works for one person is not 100% guaranteed to work for another. So, if you started the DASH diet to help you with your hypertension and it's not bringing your numbers down into the range that the doctor wants them to be in, then you should switch to another diet that helps with that condition such as Weight Watchers.

Weight Watchers can help lower blood pressure in some people that struggle on other diets. Each diet is unique - just like you are - so if you try one and you don't find the success that you're looking for, don't give up.

Just stop that one and try another. With all of the healthy diets that are available, you're sure to find one that will work for you. You might even want to switch up diet meal plans throughout the week!

It's perfectly acceptable to try two or even more diet meal plans. For example, you might adhere to a vegetarian diet three days a week, follow a Mediterranean diet two days, and the other two days, pursue the DASH diet or Weight Watchers if you'd like to work with that.

For more information about products that can support you on your Journey to Weight loss, & Amazing health visit:

SakuraNutraceuticals.com

Supplementing Your Diet Success

Chapter 10

As you go on this wellness journey in the coming year, and you find a nutritional plan you can pursue as well as an activity schedule that agrees with you, you'll want to supplement your diet with anything that helps you succeed.

Be Careful with Actual Supplements

When you're using a diet that addresses complete health concerns, you might be put on medications to help you succeed if your doctor feels you need them. You have to be careful about what you eat or use in conjunction with them.

For example, if you're on cholesterol medication, it might be wise to avoid eating grapefruit as part of your diet. You're going to read lots of conflicting advice about supplements, too.

Even natural supplements can be touted by one professional (such as Dr. Oz promoting the use of green coffee bean extract) and discouraged by other leaders in the dietary field as dangerous. Find out what your doctor recommends based on your health panel as well as disease history that your parents and grandparents suffered so that you prevent future issues.

Almost all experts *will* recommend that you try to get your nutritional value from real foods, not supplements.
No one should live on a diet of diet soda, processed foods and a handful of pills each day. That's not healthy for you.

Rewards Versus Self Care

Don't forget to supplement your journey with an ample supply of nurturing and pampering for yourself along the way. It doesn't always have to be expensive items like massages or mani/pedis.

You can do little things like giving yourself extra time to relax and read a book, or using an at home face mask to spoil yourself and keep you feeling good as you make major life changes to your physical body.
Keep yourself motivated with books and blogs that inspire you and tune out of disparaging remarks on social media or news stories that tend to get you depressed.

Most years, you've probably searched for that one perfect diet that's going to melt off the pounds and have you squeezing into a size 6 dress in 24 hours. It's time to adopt a healthy way of life – something that benefits you from a total wellness point of view.

Slam the door shut on unrealistic expectations, be willing to switch things up and be unconventional when it comes to planning your meals and getting enough exercise – and never let anyone else pressure you into harming your body through extreme weight loss measures that set you up for failure.

New Year's Road Map

Introduction

Have you ever made a New Year's resolution to lose weight and get fit and NOT followed through? Don't feel bad if you have, in fact nearly all New Year's fitness resolutions to get in great shape get abandoned not long after they are begun. I should know I've certainly been there and experienced the same sense of let-down myself.

The good news is that it doesn't have to be that way. Follow the ideas in this Guide and take action to implement them and this can be the year that sees a new you - an ideal lean and healthy you - emerge. I've used them successfully and seen them totally transform lives for the better.

They work as long as you WORK them!

You may be wondering if it's worth the effort. After all, for most of us, while getting into shape is rewarding it's often not easy. I'd argue, if you want a really high, extreme quality of life being fit isn't a WANT, but a NEED.

Here's a few reasons why, to ponder before you begin. I hope they'll help motivate you.

You Will Be MUCH More Attractive

Let's face it, a big part of getting fit is its visual appeal. If we are married, in a relationship or single it's always nice to know we look good isn't it? Being in shape not only sends out the right message about who we are externally, but for those who think about it for a minute it also tells a compelling story about who we are internally.

The type of person who cares about themselves, who has self-discipline and is far from lazy. These qualities are universally attractive. Making yourself more attractive for the New Year and beyond is a great reason to take fitness seriously.

You Will Become Healthier, Fast

Our health is our true wealth. Cutting down our body fat, getting in better cardiovascular shape and making smart diet changes will do wonders for our health. Barring any accidents these moves are nearly certain to add years to your life. They are certain to add quality of life either way.

Your Energy Levels Will Sky Rocket

Having more abundant energy stores carries over into nearly every area in our lives. This means being more productive at work without having to get strung out on four cups of coffee ever morning, to being able to get back into that old sport you love, to being able to play with the kids without needing to take a nap on the couch. Believe me, the important people in your life will appreciate the difference nearly as much as you do!

You Will Beat Depression

Now you may not be suffering from feeling down often, but the hard truth is that many out of shape people do. Getting fit is the best cure for melancholy! Forget taking drugs or mumbo jumbo therapy - carving out a new fit you for the New Year is quite likely to chase depression away for good. Try it and see. These are much closer to NEEDS than WANTS, aren't they? There's plenty more too, these are just some of the more common things that come to mind. Now, Let's get you Fit for the New Year!

Why Most
New Year's Resolutions Fail
Chapter 1

If the statistics can be believed (and they probably can) somewhere in the neighborhood of 88% of New Year's Resolutions are given up on after a few weeks.

A smart bet would be that the vast majority of these New Year resolution false starts and stumbles are broadly speaking, health related ranging from fat loss to quitting smoking and everywhere in between.

Which brings us to the next big question... Why do most New Year's Resolutions Fail?

Knowing some of the big reasons why they fail gives us an idea of what to watch out for when it comes to making sure our New Year's fitness resolutions are an absolute blinding success.

Let's see...

Putting Too Much on One Plate

Now I don't mean that literally in how much food you are eating in this case (though that may be true too!) what we're looking at is having too many Resolutions that target too many areas of life.

Big changes require big focus. If you NEED to lose weight and get more fit for the reasons, we have already discussed make getting fit a priority. Worry about getting that raise at work, learning a new language and some of the other things you may want to do after you have accomplished this important milestone.

The upside of getting fit first is that your new found confidence, energy and self-discipline will make your future goals MUCH easier to achieve. Fitness can be the foundation of the new you!

No Accountability

Often New Year's Resolutions enter the land of pipe dreams, because we leave no one accountable to them but ourselves. If this was enough most coaches and motivational speakers would be on the unemployment line. Human nature dictates that we are much more geared towards accomplishing our dreams when we let others who are important to us know about our plan and they hold us accountable to them. Even having online support through forums and discussion groups on fitness can be a huge help. Having no accountability beyond yourself is setting yourself up to fail.

An Unwillingness to Try New Things

If you keep doing the same old things there's no doubt you will continue getting the same old results. This is a unbreakable rule which requires that we step out of our comfort zones, sometimes radically, to see dramatic change in our lives.

Since you are taking the time to read this Guide, I'm very confident you are open minded enough to consider and try new things to get the body and health you deserve. Congratulations on delivering a blow to this foe of New Year's fitness resolutions already!

Thinking there is an "Easy" Way to Get Fit

Losing ugly body fat and getting your dream body to become a reality isn't easy, despite what supplement hustlers and infomercials may try to sell you.

It requires hard work, sweat and dedication. Smart tips and insider information, like you will find in this Guide and elsewhere, can and will help, but please don't think it will be "easy". Hardly anything worthwhile in life ever is. This also means when you do succeed you will have every right to be proud of your hard-earned accomplishments. This alone can be worth the price of admission!

Now that you are better prepared to know what negative elements to be on the lookout for let's dig into our program!

For more information about products that can support you on your Journey to Weight loss, & Amazing health visit:

SakuraNutraceuticals.com

The Secret to Establishing New Healthy Habits

Chapter 2

Are your habits acting like a strait jacket keeping you fat and unhappy?

What if you were able to install NEW habits - ones that made your goals easier to achieve, habits that made your body and your lifestyle more in tune with who and what you want to be?

Learning how to establish new healthy habits is a secret that can be the deciding factor in achieving your New Year's fitness resolutions and beyond. Once you get the process down, and it's not hard, you will possess a awesome new power for self-change that can totally transform your life.

Here's how it works...

Set Your Goal

Pick a small achievable goal that fits into the bigger picture of the lifestyle change you are working for, Try not to be both specific and also not too broad.

For example, "running four days a week" is a goal which works much better with this method than "eating breakfast every day, going to the gym and getting eight hours sleep."

Those are all good goals, but breaking them down into smaller pieces and working on them one by one is a much more successful approach here.

Establish a Trigger

You can think of your "trigger" as an action that signals for you to begin your new habit. This is an important part of why the method works psychologically. Continuing with running as our example a trigger could be drinking a glass of green tea or coffee every day before you immediately run.

Your trigger will stay the same as long as you work with your new habit. Many people are more visually orientated, in which case something as simple as laying your running gear out each day before work could act as a trigger to run when you return home. Experiment and see which type of trigger works best for you.

Keep it as Fun as Possible

If there's any way you can spice up your new healthy habit to make it more fun and exciting, do it! The more pleasure you can keep associated with it (or pain with NOT doing it) the better. This can be as simple as always listening to music you love while exercising or seasoning the healthy food well to make sure it consistently tastes outstanding.

Don't Stop

Skipping doing what you need to do with your new habit before it sets in will take you back to step one. It's essential you force yourself to do it for these early days even if it seems uncomfortable.

Remember, the nature of our minds is to strongly resist even positive change and to try to keep us in our comfort zone.

Which is the last place we want to be when getting ourselves into the best shape of our lives!

21 Days is the Target

Most experts agree it takes roughly 21 days for a habit to be established. After that we can expect our "inner selves" to start working with us, not against us. If you can keep it going that long, which I know you can, things will become much easier. After that pick a new healthy habit and repeat!

Have you picked a new fitness habit to get started with? I hope so!

New Year Diet Tips That Work

Chapter 3

When it comes to losing fat in the New Year almost nothing is as important as diet and you know what? Nearly every diet on the market today is probably much better than following your everyday diet that has led you to be overweight and out of shape.

This is the real reason why you hear about new "break-through" diets all the time. The people who design and market them realize they will cause people to lose weight as long as they break them out of their current over-eating habits.

Now this doesn't mean some perform better than others, they certainly do. Also some of the more radical approaches are best suited to smaller groups of people who just "click" with their dietary approach better than others.

So for New Year diet suggestions, rather than promote to you one diet over another it may be much more fruitful to share some broader weight loss tips that can get the ball rolling in the right direction while you explore and find a plan that best fits your own individual needs and desires.

You may even find, like many people I consult, that these tips alone are more than enough to get your eating habits in order. That buying and studying a 400-page diet book is an unnecessary chore and you're meeting your weight loss goals by keeping it simple and self-disciplined! Try them along with the rest of our advice in this Guide and prepare for a lean new you this New Year!

Throw Out the Junk Food

If it's in your cabinets the chances of you eating it are much, much higher than if you only had healthy food in your home isn't it? So, grab a garbage bag and throw those temptations away if you plan on getting lean. Hard advice for sure, but radical problems require radical solutions! This tip alone has saved many from emotional eating and junk food "relapse".

Eat Small but Frequent Meals

Cutting your daily calories while not putting your metabolism into starvation mode isn't as difficult as it may at first sound. Simply cut your calorie intake by 25% (or more) and divide this over five or six meals. If you are unsure about your daily calorie intake pick up one of the widely available calories counting books and copy down everything you eat and drink over a 24-hour period.

And everything means EVERYTHING. Cut this by 25% at first and continue cutting calories until you hit the magic number where you are losing weight every week on the scale. The frequent meals will make sure your metabolism stays high.

Don't Drink Calories

No soda and no juice. Beyond protein shakes you should not be drinking any calories at all. Water, green tea (without sugar) and diet soda are all your new "go to" choices.

Make Protein King

Most overweight people eat WAY too many carbohydrates. This is why low and no carb diets work so well. Cut your carbs as much as possible and replace them with protein and vegetables. Whenever you hit a plateau losing weight it's not a bad idea to cut carbs further!

Plan and Cook Your Meals in Advance

Succeeding with your New Year's fat loss program requires planning and preparation. Having a good idea of what you will be eating every day before it begins is setting yourself up to achieve your dreams. Even better is cooking a few easy meals like lunches for work in advance. If not, you are at the mercy of external factors which can (and will) sabotage your diet quickly and without mercy!

These tips aren't complicated and they work. Once they are in place you may choose to expand your diet plan or you may not. Either way you can expect to be shedding more weight and getting more fit every single week. Sounds good doesn't it!

A New Year's Exercise Plan You Can Stick With

Chapter 4

Now for the fun stuff! While most of us find dieting to be a bit (or much more than a bit) of a chore, a fitness routine is something that can become the highlight of your day once you get into the swing of things. Really, there's few things as satisfying as seeing your strength rise as you stick with a good exercise plan. The weights don't lie and as you progress it's near impossible not to have your sense of wellbeing and self-worth rise along with the heavier dumbbells and barbells!

For our get fit for the New Year plan we're going to keep it simple. There's no complicated moves or exercises. If you do see something you are unfamiliar with a YouTube or Google search is sure to answer any questions of form.

For complete beginners ask a friend to hit the gym or the garage with you one day to help walk you through it. Or even schedule one or two sessions with a personal trainer to catch you up to speed though I doubt that's necessary for 99.9% of our readers!

We'll be training three non-consecutive days a week, split into A workouts and B workouts.

On week 1 we will do our A Workout on Monday and Friday and B workout on Wednesday.

On week 2 we reverse the days and do our B Workout on Monday and Friday and B workout on Wednesday.

This somewhat abbreviated schedule compared to what you have likely read in fitness or bodybuilding magazines is perfect for cutting fat, getting toned and building strength. There's no fear of over training, which is something that can cause your New Year's weight loss to grind to a standstill.

All exercises should be done with a weight that causes you to fail with your last set. If you make your final rep goal increase the weight in your next session. Don't forget to keep a long to make sure you keep moving forward!

Workout A

* Dumbbell Bench Presses. 4 sets of 8 reps.
* Lat Pull Down. 4 sets of 8 reps. If you are strong enough sub pull ups for lat pull downs.
* Barbell Curls. 4 sets of 10 reps.
* Dumbbell or Machine Shoulder Presses. 4 sets of 12 reps.
* Crunches. 4 sets to failure.

Workout B

* Barbell Squat or Machine Leg Press. 5 sets of 12 reps.
* Barbell Stiff Leg Dead Lifts or Machine Hamstring Curls. 5 sets of 12 reps.
* Seated Calf Raises. 4 sets of 12 reps.
* Dumbbell Shrugs. 4 Sets of 8 reps.
* Leg or Knee Lifts for Lower Abs. 3 sets to failure.

And that's it!

You can see on Week 1 we will be training our upper body twice and lower body plus some abs and our traps once.

On Week 2 we will do our lower body twice and upper body once. With our diet and cardio on point this is the perfect training program to carve out the body of our dreams.

Just be sure you train like you mean it! Intensity is key to your success and sleep walking your way through your program can't be expected to do much good at all can it?

IF you give 100% real miracles can and will happen.

For more information about products that can support you on your Journey to Weight loss, & Amazing health visit:

SakuraNutraceuticals.com

The Truth About Cardio

Chapter 5

Have you seen many fat marathon runners?

Overweight sprinters?

How about flabby guys or girls who bike ride obsessively?

No, you probably haven't. And neither have I. The reason being despite what some fitness "experts" may try to push in order to sell an "easier" program, is that cardio works wonders in getting one lean and healthy. Very few people you see who are in AWESOME shape got that way without doing cardio. All the rest put in the work and paid in sweat to get their dream bodies. If you'd like to unveil the best you possible for the New Year you will have to to also!

So what's the best approach towards Cardio for losing weight? Here are some of the secrets...

Both Long Distance Low Intensity and High Intensity Interval Cardio Can Work Well.

Weight loss cardio advocates usually fall into one of two camps. The first suggest long distance cardio at a low or moderate intensity. This could be power walking, jogging or biking for an hour a day, five or six days a week.

The other camp pushes very intense, but short cardio plans with things like hill sprints, rowing machine sessions and so on. There's no surprise, really, in that each method works well. Which you choose is more a matter of first your initial fitness level (the less fit you are the more appropriate low intensity cardio is) and your personal taste. Choose the one you enjoy more and is less of a strain sticking to.

Train Five or Six Days a Week

With cardio the more often you train the better, Do at least five days. Six is even better if your schedule allows.

Fasted Cardio Burns Fat Fast

The best time to do cardio to lose body fat most efficiently is in a fasted state. For most of us the most practical time to do this is first thing in the morning after not eating for our eight or more hours of sleep. This is a trick discovered by professional bodybuilders looking for every advantage in contest preparation. It can speed up your fat loss by 25% or more!

Don't Be Afraid to Mix Up Your Cardio Choices

Personally, I can relate to the people who find cardio a bit boring. A nice way to fight this (after being sure to have a MP3 player with a kick ass play list) is to cycle through a few different cardio choices. On Monday and Wednesday, I run on the treadmill at the gym, on Tuesday and Thursday I bike ride in my neighborhood and Saturday is dedicated to high intensity rowing machine work. This can keep things much fresher and more fun.

Stay Safe

Never launch a cardio session without a ten-minute stretching session first. The last thing you want is a New Year's pulled hamstring or worse to slow down your fat loss momentum. Think of stretching as your body's insurance policy. Never neglect it. Believe me. I learned this lesson the hard way!

Diet, exercise and now cardio. You've earned your degree in the three courses of New Year's fat loss! Congratulations.

Lifestyle Changes that Make the Difference

Chapter 6

We've gone over a great deal of the nuts and bolts of how you can and will get fit for the New Year. Will you be able to STAY fit once you put in all the time and hard and smart work?

The answer to that very important question rests on whether you are able to make the positive lifestyle changes that support the fit new you rather than work against you.

Over the years, I have been able to identify some of the most common lifestyle changes that friends and clients have had to master before they were able to set their new levels of fitness in stone and not relapse back into their old ways. You have a HUGE head start knowing what to look out for as you make your New Year's weight loss goals solid and real.

Avoid the Negative Few Who Would See You Fail

There's an element of person who feels VERY threatened by those who are able to work at positive self-change - and especially at something like weight loss. Rather than asking how you were able to cut fat and trying it themselves they'd rather put temptation after temptation in front of you until you fall off track.

Do they do this consciously? Who knows, but it happens and happens frequently.

If staying lean, healthy and fit is important to you a vital lifestyle change is to avoid spending too much time around this type of influence. They will only drag you down.

Get Off the Couch and Have Fun

Your new body shouldn't just be for show. As you get in better and better shape make sure you have fun using it! This will reinforce the idea that the new you is worth the work and sacrifices. Play that old or new sport you love, going dancing or take the kids for an active day at the beach. All these things should be taking the place of television and video games more and more until NOT being fit becomes unthinkable.

Share What You Know

A self-help genius once said that the best way to keep what you have is to teach it to others. Do you have friends and loved ones who could use a bit of motivation or could benefit from the knowledge you have picked up from this Guide and elsewhere? Why not teach or train them? Who knows in the future this could even turn into a new hobby or a part- or full-time way to make a living? Stranger things have happened that's for sure.

Don't underestimate the power of these three lifestyle shifts. They may seem minor, but they are anything but. In fact, they could be the deciding factor on how you look and feel two, five, ten years from now and beyond.

Being lean, attractive and healthy isn't a set of moves and diet choices. It's a way of life. A way of life that's probably one of the most rewarding things that you could ever dedicate your time and effort to. Give it your all!

Keeping Your Mind Right The Inner Game of Getting fit

Chapter 7

Just about every top athlete would tell you, if you asked, that 90% of the physical game is mental.

Our minds command our bodies ultimately and staying on point with our weight loss goals has MUCH more to do with what's going on inside our heads than not. It's only the rarest situation where our body will fail us in training and leave us with an injury. Taking the time to train safe largely prevents this.

On the other hand, situations where a person trying to lose weight sees their minds fail resulting in skipped workouts or junk food eating binges are much, much more common.

Thankfully. there're a few simple things we can do to develop our "Inner Game" of fitness. These tips can make an ally of our minds rather than an enemy!

Use Positive Visualizations

Our subconscious mind has great difficulty separating what we image from what has actually occurred or is occurring. This trait can be harmful, but when we harness it and use it to our advantage it can also be pure magic. How can we do this? Sit comfortably with eyes shut. In your mind imagine how you will look lean and fit in the New Year.

After around five minutes move on to yourself performing in the gym powerfully and dynamically.

After a few minutes more move back to seeing yourself again lean and fit. In total this can be worked on for ten or fifteen minutes a day as many days as you are able. Watch the wonders ensue.

Practice Affirmations to Build Confidence

Think of affirmations as an approach to the subconscious audibly like visualizations are visually. They pay off just as much. When both these methods are used, they complement each other perfectly. How do affirmations work? Take a short positive set of statements and repeat it to yourself, out loud in the morning and evening. An example: "I am healthy, fit and happy". Always state things in the present terms with "I am" and your goals stated as if already achieved. Never use "I want" or " I am not". The way the mind works these things don't sink in nearly as well.

When Stressed Breathe DEEPLY

Breathing influences the mind. When you become stressed about your ability to achieve your New Year's fitness goals, or anything else really, breathe deeply. Here's a traditional "calming" breathing technique used in yoga. It's worked for over a thousand years. Inhale for a count of four. Hold your breath for a count of eight. Exhale for a count of twelve while you imagine your bad thoughts leaving with your breath. Repeat twenty times or until you feel yourself relax.

Don't be surprised if you feel yourself developing more mental focus and energy throughout the day as you do the calming breath more frequently. These positive side effects come with the territory.

There's an inner and outer game to most things worth doing in life fat loss and fitness included.

Now you're armed with the skill to become a champion of your New Year's weight loss inner game will you use it? I hope so, because this is one game that s definitely worth winning.

For more information about products that can support you on your Journey to Weight loss, & Amazing health visit:

SakuraNutraceuticals.com

Staying on Course the Whole Year and Beyond

Chapter 8

We've touched on lifestyle changes we need to make to protect our fitness choices. Now it's time to explore a few other areas that will help us stay on course for our New Year and beyond. Because this WILL be the year we put on and off fitness efforts to an end for good won't it? The idea is to take off the weight and keep it off. And I'm going to give you every tool and trick I know of to make that idea a success!

Schedule Regular Fitness Times

Just like you get up on time five days a week (or more) to go to school or work, you should do the same for your fitness training if you want to stay on course for the long term. Sticking with the same time incorporates what we have learned in our Chapter on Habits to our advantage. Having it set that training is an everyday part of life like going to work makes losing our gains next to impossible. I have close friends who have stuck with this tip for years and made fitness transformations that should be on television they are so amazing. Persistence pays.

Review Your Progress

Keeping a photo album, either shirtless in shorts (for guys) or in bathing suits (for women) starting at day one with updates every month over the years gives a clear, solid picture of why staying on course is so vital. Whenever you feel the temptation to be lazy or over indulge head to the closet and open to day one. Ask yourself if you would like to go back there, or worse? I'm betting that junk food will have lost its appeal pretty quickly.

Ignore Training and Diet Fads

There are certainly fitness sources that provide valuable, actionable and useful information free from hype and over-self-interest. I would like to think I am one of them. There are also fitness sources that will try to sell you snake oil and useless programs just to make a buck. These are best ignored as they can distract you from what works and sometimes even cause injury. Buck the trends and keep things simple. Only accept advice from those who have earned your trust.

Remember MORE is Always Possible

Don't let your successes seem like the end of the road.

There are always new goals that can be set and accomplished that can bring you even more excitement and joy.

Your lean now, but haven't you always wanted six pack abs? Well figure out how to get them and work towards it! Or how about doing 25 pull ups for those who like strength goals? Or 100 pushups without stopping? Or running a marathon? If setting big new fitness goals helps motivate you keep doing it and accomplish them one by one. Before you know it, you may have a fitness resume fit for an award-winning auto biography!

Thinking of your New Year's weight loss resolution as a starting point for a new active healthy life is where it's at. We all had to start somewhere. The finish line is something we should NEVER set. The future should always be exciting and something we look forward to!

Take Action - Build a New YOU for the New Year

Chapter 9

You can have the best information on weight loss in the world, a membership to an A class gym and one of the coaches from television's "The Biggest Loser" as your success coach, but without the willingness to take action what is it all worth?

Nothing

If you are truly serious about building a new YOU for the New Year you have to stop being a person who JUST reads about it. Or talks about it. Or thinks about it. Or PLANS to do it. You NEED to be the type of person who uses fat loss knowledge as fuel and inspiration and who takes swift action to put it to good use.

Taking action is the final key to making sure you succeed with your New Year's weight loss goals and beyond! Otherwise, things will stay the same. If not become worse. It's a truth that can't be escaped.

Don't forget...

ACTION is the Way to Success

Everything here in our Guide from positive thinking to the diet and exercise plans are basically worthless if they aren't applied. They all need to be put into effect through you taking ACTION for their benefits to be felt and seen. Your new body will be built through action not through talking, reading or thinking alone. If getting lean didn't require work there would be a lot more fantastic looking people in the world.

Many overweight and out of shape people have whole libraries full of fitness books and hard drives packed with weight loss guides. They never lose a pound because they never act on the things they've read. Don't be one of these people.

Today is Better than Tomorrow

Many good intentioned people spend months and even years putting off their efforts into getting into shape until "tomorrow". Sadly, this tomorrow keeps being postponed again and again. Meanwhile, the pounds continue to pack on and their quality of life stays far removed from what it could be. Live up to your full potential. Don't wait for the perfect conditions to begin. They may never come. Start today, regardless. Tomorrow may never come.

Keep Moving Forward

Stasis is the enemy of getting fit. Once you get started do everything in your power to keep moving forward. The small actions you take every day are a continuation of your important decision to get started. These little victories will add up until you see the dream you staring back in the mirror one day. You can bet on it.

Now the ball is in your court. You've taken the time to acquire and read our Guide. You've committed to building a lean, fit and healthy New You for the New Year. All that's left is to get things started for real in the real world. Make today the first day of the rest of your life. I know you can do it and I can hardly wait to hear about your successes big and small. This is the New Year where it all changes for the better. Can you feel it too?

BONUS
How to Enjoy the Holidays WITHOUT Packing on Pounds!

The Holidays need to be treated with respect if we hope to not torpedo our weight loss goals!

For many people these few weeks add up to complete diet disaster. For a quick example, did you know Americans on average gain seven pounds between Thanksgiving in November and New Year's Day? This is a terrible statistic considering how difficult many find it to shed pounds.

Wishing for a healthier way to celebrate the Holidays? Read on and find out how you can still have fun without giving yourself a spare tire around the waist for Christmas!

Stay Hydrated

The more water you drink the less calories you will eat. Staying hydrated is a sure way to not over indulge on food because of false "hunger" signals. Water is your calorie less, health providing friend. Drink lots of it.

Fill Up on Protein

There's no need to skip the holiday meals with friends and family. Just make sure to focus on eating protein. Think a little extra turkey or ham over potatoes and rice. More carbs with less activity is a sure way to get fat. Protein, on the other hand, is much more forgiving.

Drink in Moderation

Alcohol binges on New Year's Eve can really be a mess if you are drinking calorie heavy beer and mixed drinks. Drink moderately and choose less harmful options when you can. You can still have fun while not torching your physique believe me!

Amp Up the Cardio

Don't skip workout sessions during the Holidays. Why not up the intensity instead? You will surely have the time to get your cardio in and this can be a pretty effective counter measure should you stumble and over eat a bit. Even if you can only manage a half session or the gym is closed and you run at home, anything is better than doing NOTHING,

Try Adding in Fast Days

Yes, fasting works. Why not add in a "fast" day where you drink only calorie less liquids for every day where you broke your diet? This has been shown to be both safe and effective. You may even decide to give fasting a shot during your normal schedule too. If you do be sure to check out an Intermittent Fasting Guide or book to get yourself caught up to speed.

Have a Holiday Success Coach

Sign up a friend, family member or significant other as your Holiday Success Coach. Their job is to keep watch what goes on your plate and give you a scowl should you get out of hand. Also encouraging you to workout is part of the job position. Be sure to reward them with a great Christmas gift and a drink or two on New Year's!

It's not the end of the world if you put on a pound or two over the holidays. If you keep these tips in mind and apply them the worst excesses can be avoided. This sets you up perfectly for having the best fitness year of your life! There's no better gift you can give yourself for the New Year and beyond.

For more information about products that can support you on your Journey to Weight loss, & Amazing health visit:

SakuraNutraceuticals.com

Secrets of Working with Weights

Introduction

Fitness and strength building trends can be a dime a dozen. Those of us who have had a glimpse behind the fitness industry scenes have often seen firsthand what motivates its gurus. It is not how to help people get fit, fast or experience vibrant health, but how to shovel morecash into their bank accounts.

What if there were a proven fitness method, that didn't require any special equipment, no gym membership or supplement and diet options were strictly your own decision?

This would-be bad news for the health and fitness profiteers and great news for you wouldn't it?

Welcome to Bodyweight Training

This method holds all these qualities and more. By the time you are through with this guide you will have all the information you need to build a new ripped and powerful you and you can do it all in your living room or backyard! Exciting isn't it? When you see the end results you will be even more excited!

Read on and you'll find...

- Bodyweight Training is a Completely New Challenge. If you have any sort of gym experience you may become one of the many who is excited to realize what an exciting new challenge Bodyweight Training can be. No more waiting for someone to spot you while you bench press, or messing around on the latest fitness machine atthe gym.

- Instead, you'll be cranking out pushups and hitting the pull up bar in the door way. This can be quite refreshing trust me!

- Bodyweight Training Torches Body Fat. Missing your abs? Follow a Bodyweight Training only program and you'll find your missing six pack in no time. Many of usget ultra-shredded via Bodyweight Training only, with only minimal cardio.

- Bodyweight Training Heals Injuries and Builds Flexibility. Pounding the weights for year after year oftenleaves us with a laundry list of unhealed injuries. Many will quickly heal up once we switch our training protocol and focus on Bodyweight Training alone. On top of this the flexibility benefits can be compared to an original Bodyweight Training method - yoga (which was originallyused by Indian warriors as a conditioning method!)

- Bodyweight Training Supercharges Endurance. Kiss thetreadmill goodbye. High rep Bodyweight Training will build real endurance WHILE you build great looking muscle!

- Bodyweight Training Gets You Fit On A Budget. Apart from some instruction (which you are reading right now)you can train without any added expense at all. Need tosave money? Now you can get fit without going near a gym unless you choose too.

- Bodyweight Training Builds Toughness. Truth be told, the toughest guys in the world train following BodyweightTraining almost exclusively.

- Military elite units and special forces, boxers, wrestlers and mixed martial artists - eveninmates in the world's most dangerous prisons. Bodyweight Training will make you fit, healthy and toughtoo!

- Well let's get into it, I'm very happy to have you here reading our guide, where I'll do my best to open your eyes to a whole new approach to achieving your fitnessgoals. Be prepared to think a bit out of the box and youmay never want to lift a weight again. The best body ofyour life awaits

The Secret History of Bodyweight Training

Chapter 1

I've already touched on the fact that the majority of the fitness "powers that be" would prefer that Bodyweight Training were brushed over and ignored in favor of much less potent conditioning ideas. The inarguable fact is that no other strength and conditioning method has such a shining history of effectiveness. Going all the way back to ancient times and lasting until today.

Don't take my word for it. Here's some historicalhighlights of Bodyweight Training...

- The Indian Wrestling Cults. Did you know Indian wrestling as a sport (and near religion) goes back thousands of years? Approaching modern MMA in its mix of grappling and striking, Indian wrestlers developed extensive libraries of Bodyweight Training exercises, some revived in the last decade or so outside of India likethe Hindu pushup and Hindu squat which we will touch on later in our guide. The physical prowess of Indian wrestlers is legendary with well documented programs that included over 500 pushups and 1000 squats a day, six days a week!

- The Spartan Warriors. If you've ever seen a statue or painting of a Spartan warrior you will probably have seenthat the movie "300" was right on the mark with their depiction of the Spartan physique. The Spartans lifted noweights, but trained using advanced Bodyweight Trainingmethods which left them with a still lasting reputation of being some of the finest physical specimen to ever walk the earth.

- The Roman Gladiator. A distant cousin of the Spartan,Roman Gladiators employed similar training programs brought to them from the Greeks. Their results were equally impressive.

- Charles Atlas and the American Physical Culturalists. The idea of building a healthy, great looking and powerfulbody first reignited in modern days at the start of the 1900's. Probably the most popular and well known of these fitness enthusiasts was the legendary Charles Atlas.Charles, along with most of his contemporaries, were dedicated Bodyweight Training advocates and built insanely well developed and athletically capable bodies. Google Charles Atlas, Earle Liederman, Jack Lalanne or other fitness gurus of their era and marvel at what theywere able to achieve minus weights, anabolic steroids, supplements or even advanced diet ideas!

- Modern Military Spec Ops. From the American Navy Seals to the British RAF and every special force group in between has been built on a foundation of pushups, pull ups, crunches and so on. Very few indulge in much weight training. Can anyone really deny their high level ofconditioning and life and death level of true functional fitness?

- Matt Furey and the New Breed of Bodyweight Training. In the early 2000's a somewhat over the top fitness coach and author is credited by most as bringing back Bodyweight Training to the forefront of discussion and reviving a whole arsenal of lost exercises. Furey opened these doors and deserves more credit than he sometimes receives.

Now it should be clear you are about to follow in some very legendary footsteps when you dive into BodyweightTraining.

Are you ready to carry on this proud fitness tradition? I think you absolutely have what it takes.

Time to move forward!

For more information about products that can support you on your Journey to Weight loss, & Amazing health visit:

SakuraNutraceuticals.com

First Things First -Stretching & Warming Up

Chapter 2

No matter what type of training we engage in safety should always come first. Bodyweight training is no exception to this golden rule. After all, when injured we can hardly train at all can we? So, paying close attentionto things like warming up and stretching before our training sessions ultimately leads us to getting stronger and fitter in no time at all. Pay close attention to this chapter. My suggestions are simple, but they should notbe skipped or glossed over, trust me!

Bodyweight Training Warm Ups

Warming up for Bodyweight Training is much less complicated than some of the schemes you may be used to if you have done much weight lifting. Our goal is to getthe blood flowing and raise our temperature before we doour light stretching. This helps make us more limber for our stretches and further reduces our chance of injury.

How you choose to do this is really a matter of personal choice, but I suggest you aim for the ten-minute mark. A brisk walk or jog is what I choose to do most often, but if you prefer using the bike or a rowing machine that's fine too. Many of my friends who are involved in combat sports go old school and jump rope or hit the punching heavy bag.

As long as we accomplish the goal of getting our blood circulating and temperature rising without overdoing it feel free to choose which ever cardio methodyou prefer.

Stretching Tips and Ideas

Again, warming up and stretching is a must before every workout session. After your ten-minute warm up another ten minutes of stretching unless you have special needs to address will get the job done effectively.

- Don't Bounce in Your Stretches. Stretch calmly and witha slow and controlled effort. This will not only give you the best results, but all will avoid tearing any tight muscles. We are stretching to prevent injury NOT causeinjury!

- Control Your Breathing. Erratic breathing can detract from the benefits of stretching. Exhale into your stretch and continue breathing full deep breaths as you maintainyour stretch.

- The Magic Thirty. Hold your stretches for thirty seconds. Research has shown this is the amount of timethat offers the most benefit for the athlete.

- Never Stretch into Pain. Stretching should NOT hurt. "No pain - no gain" may apply to other areas of training.It never, ever applies to stretching! Please don't ignore this tip.

- Consider having a go at Yoga. Yoga can be a really awesome compliment to Bodyweight Training. The false impression that yoga is just for women is losing more ground every day, with Football and Rugby players, alongwith mixed martial artists all singing the praises of this ancient art form. Yoga can help you experience real health benefits along with flexibility.

- Combined with Bodyweight Training you can truly build the ideal body inthe privacy of your own home with no equipment neededat all.

Between warming up and stretching you'll be ready to train in twenty minutes. Give this twenty minute the same attention you pay to the rest of your training andyour body will thank you. It goes a long way towards becoming near injury proof!

The Miracle of The Pushup & Dips

A solid hard chest, horse shoe triceps and ripped abs too. Sky rocketing upper body power. Even bragging rights among friends. The pushup and its cousin the bodyweight dip offer all this and much more. If you had to choose only two exercises to perform this would be the first half (the second being pull ups of course!)

Exploring the Pushup

Used everywhere from the school yard, to the gym and dojo to the sand and dirt of special forces training campsthe push up is rightly beloved as one of the simplest andbest exercises we could ever perform. Embrace it.

Here's some pushup tips to keep in mind

Always use Proper Pushup Form. Many of us have picked up bad habits in the way we execute our pushups over the years. Here's proper pushup form:

1. Keep yourself stiff and tight - including your abs.
2. Elbows at a forty-five-degree angle at the sides of your body.
3. Take a breath as you lower your chest to the floor.
4. Exhale as you press up.
5. Repeat.

- Engage your Mind while doing Pushups. It's helpful tovisualize your palms exploding through the floor while doing your pushups as a means to building more explosive power.

- Raise your Feet for a Upper Chest Emphasis. Place yourfeet on a chair, bed or better yet a inflatable exercise ballto focus the emphasis of the pushup more greatly on the upper chest and shoulders. This can help develop a morepleasing physique by most accounts.

- Don't be Frightened to go High Volume. It's not uncommon for Bodyweight Training enthusiasts to do 100, 250 or even 500 pushups every few days. Ignore those who cry about "over training" from Bodyweight training. This has proven to give fantastic results and isexactly the method used in modern military - and in prisons too, to build seriously hard and strong muscle!

Dynamic Dipping

After pushups our next powerful chest, triceps and really total upper body builder is the dip. How we choose to do dips depends on our strength levels, conditioning and what we have in our surroundings to perform our dips on.

- Parallel Bar Dips. The traditional dip that requires the most starting strength to begin training with. With your hands on two bars (or handles) you dip your entire bodyand press it back up using your upper body power. Manyschool yards have parallel bars to dip from allowing you to train for free in the sun while forging a mighty upper body.

- Chair Dips. Putting your hands on a chair behind your back while your legs are extended and heels resting on asecond chair (your body should be roughly "L" shaped) this offers a much easier dip version for those who findfull dips too difficult.

- The Atlas Dip. My personal favorite of the dips taken from the Golden Age strong man and physical culture guru Charles Atlas. Two chairs are placed in front of you about 20 inches apart depending on how wide your shoulders are. Place a hand on each chair seat while yourbody is extended behind you, feet on the floor. Perform pushups between the chairs. Atlas suggested way back in1922 for his students to do at least 200 a day, working their way up to what he did - 500!

This is a really superb exercise many modern trainers aren't aware of. It can be a game changer in building a great looking chest, shoulders and triceps too! Try it and I think you will be impressed with your results.

With this information rejoice! A new chest is now rightaround the corner!

Pull Up Power

Chapter 3

You should not consider yourself anywhere near being strong, fit or in shape if you can't do a pull up. Thanks to the modern age of "all show - no go" fitness machines we've had at least a generation of trainers doing everything they can to avoid hitting the pull up bar. Pull downs, back machines, bands, on and on and on trying to"fix" an exercise that was never broke in the first place. We all know not to fix things that aren't broke, don't we?If not we certainly should!

With that behind us many may start their Bodyweight Training journey with the need to build strength and power in their pull up ability. This will reap tremendous benefits - the more pull ups you do regularly the better you will look and feel. Ninety days of pull ups will likely leave you looking like an action movie star or superhero.

Follow these suggestions and you'll be doing sets oftwenty in no time!

- Avoid Going to Failure. In building Pull Up strength andpower it's been shown again and again it's best to avoid going to failure in sets. Always leave a rep or two in the bank. Do more sets while avoiding going to failure ratherthan blowing out all your energy on only one or two sets.Even though this may seem counter initiatory this will quickly turn into huge jumps in strength. Olympic athletes swear by this method. Try it and you will too!

- Pull with the Lats First. Pull with your back muscles first NOT your arms. Obviously, your lats being much larger muscles they possess more power and endurance than your biceps. Use this to your advantage.

- Keep Your Elbows Pointing Back and Down. This will aide you in firing your lats in the movement. Try to imageelbowing someone behind you in their stomach. Like the guy who convinced you to add this grueling exercise to your Bodyweight training sessions (just kidding!)

- Get your Chin over the Bar. There's no need to go chestto the bar like some trainers claim. Anything much beyond your chin does little to add further to your backdevelopment. Instead consider your chin going over thebar as a good solid rep.

- Lose Body Fat. The leaner you are the better your pull up ability will become. Fat people don't do many pull upsand pull up masters are very rarely (if ever) fat. When you set a goal of putting up massive numbers on the pullup bar it's good encouragement in the quest to also get lean. One drive compliments the other quite nicely!

- Switch Up Your Grips. Okay technically speaking pull ups are when your palms are facing you. Chin ups are when your palms are facing away from you. Neutral gripsare when you are using a bar that allows your palms to be facing each other. Do a few sets of each when you train upper body. This will help build your back from different angles and also do wonders for your grip strength!

There's no better feeling than being able to hop up and grab the bar pounding out easy reps of pull ups. It's a lost art even the big and strong in bodybuilding gyms are usually unable to manage.

Put in smart and steady work and you'll be leaving jaws open and fielding questions onhow you built up your new found pull up power! Feel freeto tell them about our guide.

For more information about products that can support you on your Journey to Weight loss, & Amazing health visit:

SakuraNutraceuticals.com

Wheels of Steel LegTraining Without Weights

Chapter 4

You may have heard one of the ignorant claims that it's impossible to build powerful and aesthetically pleasing looking legs without throwing half a ton on the leg press machine or squatting 500lbs. Never mind what that typeof non-stop pounding often ends up doing to the knees. Ask anyone who has power lifted or follow exclusively heavy bodybuilding leg routines for over ten years if youdon't believe me. I guarantee many mention a knee surgery or two.

The great news is that legs respond exceptionally well to high rep training Bodyweight methods. Size, strength, endurance and shapeliness are all within reach doing the following bodyweight exercises alone. You will also be much more likely to stay injury free! Can't beat that can you?

- Bodyweight Squat. The foundation of your Bodyweight leg training routine. Lock your fingers behind your head and drop glutes to the floor. Explode up. Repeat. Also called prisoner squats for their popularity behind bars these will build true explosive leg power, flexibility and endurance too. Aim for a few hundred a session. A close friend uses these as his full cardio workout and twenty tothirty minutes of Bodyweight Squats a day has left him ripped to the bone! Much cooler than running on a treadmill that's for sure.

- Bodyweight Lunges. Lunge forward with one going as low as possible. The knee of your rear leg should come close to touching the floor. Step back to standing and repeat with opposite leg. A good secondary movement tothe Bodyweight Squat that can strengthen your glutes and cut up your quads even further.

- Toe Raises. Stand on stairs or box with one leg. Raiseup on tip of your toes engaging your calf muscle. Drop down as far as possible. Repeat. When finished switch legs and do the same number of reps. Excellent calf builder where you should aim for as many reps aspossible.

- Jumping Jacks. I'm sure you remember these as a kid don't you? Use jumping jacks as both a leg builder and cardio tool. Rather than reps, set an alarm clock for a certain time and try to beat it at each session. Don't be surprised when your body fat quickly melts away as yourlower body gets more toned and stronger. Those old gymteachers in physical education class seem to have had much more actionable knowledge than they often are given credit for... further proof that in the field of strength and conditioning newer is not always better.

Sometimes falling back on old near forgotten methods represents the true cutting edge in building a new and better body!

All in all, see for yourself what a great leg workout you can get using a few fairly simple exercises, focused with power and intensity while never touching a weight or stepping on a machine. After you do, try your best not to laugh in the face of the next person sweating on the Stair Master or doing 150lb leg extensions. Once you are in on this secret and powerful fitness knowledge, I can tell you it's definitely tempting!

But don't forget we all have to start somewhere!

Back & Neck Bridges From the Wrestler's Tool Box

Chapter 5

It may not be the first thing people check out when you sun tan on the beach, but a strong lower back can save you all sorts of headaches in life. From making you less injury prone at work or protecting the spine if you engagein any hard contact sports, time spent training the lower back can be rightly thought of very much as a health insurance policy in all the best ways.

A Bodyweight Exercise from the wrestler's tool box - the Back and Neck bridge offer us the best of the best lower back builders, once again completely ignored by mainstream trainers and fitness gurus. Never use one of those dumb back extension machines ever again!

Here's some thoughts concerning the Wrestler's Bridge...

- Try to Get a First-Hand Lesson in Bridging. It's important before you try to do your first back bridge to ideally get a lesson from someone with bridging experience face to face. If this isn't possibly taking the tipsfrom this guide, read a bit further on the internet and watch some of the many YouTube demonstrations beforeyou try your first go at it. When done correctly they are more than safe, but having a clear visual lesson on the proper technique is a must just to be sure no mistakes are made.

- Start with Wall Walks. Stand with your back to a wall roughly two feet away. Arch your back and slowly and securely wall walk down with your hands continuing to arch your back. This will condition your lower back for fullfloor wrestler's bridges in a short time.

- Back Bridge Details. The wrestler's back bridge is whenyou arch your back and your bodyweight is on your palms. Hold for time.

- Neck Bridge Details. The wrestler's neck bridge is whenyou arch your back and your bodyweight in on your forehead and neck. Also hold for time.

- Shoot for Duration NOT for Reps. With bridging you areaiming to hold the bridge for longer and longer times at full extension, rather than working for reps. This builds tremendous strength, makes your stabilizer muscles powerful and even helps to develop supreme will power and force of mind. Using a small stop watch or kitchen timer is the best way to increase time under pressure without having to distract yourself counting.

- Always Stretch After Doing Bridges. It's a great habit toget into doing "toe touch" leg stretches after back bridging to make sure you are conditioning both sides of your muscles as a injury prevention measure. Take around five minutes (or more if you'd like) to engage in stretching after your back and neck bridges.

- Skip if You Have Previous Back Injuries. If you have prior lower back issues either skip the wrestler's bridgesor get your Doctor's okay before you dive in. Remembersafety always comes first!

Pushups, pull ups, back bridges. Bodyweight Training is very much akin to old school fight training. It's real hard once you get momentum

going to not feel like you'repreparing for a prize fight and that's a great thing.

Our challenges may not be in a ring, but a fighting spiritand strong and healthy body makes all of life's obstaclesmuch easier to overcome. I can tell you that much from hard earned personal experience!

For more information about products that can support you on your Journey to Weight loss, & Amazing health visit:

SakuraNutraceuticals.com

Core of Steel

Chapter 6

Bodyweight Training has huge advantages over other training methodologies in many areas. The most shiningof them is an area that's dear to nearly everyone interested in getting into great shape - developing a ripped and powerful core.

Let's be clear - no other style of training will give you six pack abs as quickly and with as extra little effort as Bodyweight Training. Bodyweight Training is the perfect storm for getting theperfect core.

There are many reasons for this - first and foremost your abs and lower back are trained in nearly all of your major training movements. Pushups, pull ups, Bodyweight squats - they all help build their target muscles groups while also as a bonus carve out your six pack. How's that for win / win? Say good bye to the endless reps on the stupid abdominalcrunch that never produced any results anyway. I doubt you'll miss it!

Here's a look at some Core Bodyweight Training exercises that shouldn't be neglected on your path to the abs of your dreams...

- The V Up. Also called by old school Bodyweight trainingenthusiasts the "Atlas sit up." Lay on your back with yourlegs fully extended and curl your upper body up while also bringing up your legs. Touch finger tips to toes. Thiscan be somewhat difficult if you are a bit out of shape - ifso, start with normal floor crunches and sit ups until a bit more core strength is developed. Just be sure to add the V ups as soon as possible they are more than worth the effort.

- Leg Raises. Hanging from a pull up bar (which will alsobuild your grip strength) raise your legs to a "L" positionusing your lower ab muscles. Beginners feel free to startby doing knee rather than full extended leg raises until more strength is built. Many fail to achieve a six or eight pack simply because they've neglected their lower abs.

- Plank. Lay in push up position. Come up on elbows andforearms keeping your body straight tightening your absas if you were about to be punched in the stomach. Holdfor time - twenty seconds in a good start, working up to sets of sixty seconds or more.

- Side Plank. Perhaps the best overall exercise for building powerful obliques. Lie on your side and come upon your elbow keeping your body tight and in a straight line, tightening your core again as if preparing for a punch to the stomach. Hold for time.

- Mountain Climbers. This is a powerful total body exercise with an emphasis on abs. It is also hugely effective as a cardio technique. Go into push up position.Press up and stay up.

- Alternate bringing knees to chest as quickly as possible. Go for time and expect to break aserious sweat. Mountain climbers are a true warrior's exercise - if you want a body that looks like something out of the movie 300 throw it all into your mountain climbers!

Ninety days of Bodyweight Training may well leave you with a bullet proof core - the type of abs no machine could ever produce.

Diet Ideas & How To Set Up Your Schedule
Chapter 7

What follows are two areas that are pretty wide open for Bodyweight Trainers to put their own personal spin on things. Diet and how to set up your schedule. I'll give you my own ideas, but your own lifestyle and individual needs may call for something a bit different.

Either way Bodyweight Training as described in this Guide will get the job done much more efficiently than any Crunch Fitness circuit of machine training ever will!

Broad but Effective Diet Ideas

Your diet is dictated by just what type of shape you are in now and what your end goals are. If you are too fat and looking to get lean obviously your diet strategy is not going to be in line with someone who is a tooth pick and looking to put on mass.

- For the Overweight. The most important thing is to establish a calorie deficit. There are many different ways to achieve this and quite a few "specialties" diet plans that will absolutely work for you to lose weight. One that fits perfectly with the minimalist approach of Bodyweight Training and is near miraculous as far as torching body fat goes is intermittent fasting.

- For those looking to Bulk Up. If you are looking to put on mass, up your calorie intake and make especially sureyou are consuming enough protein -

the building blocks of muscles. I'd suggest aiming for roughly 1 gram of protein per pound you weigh split over five or six meals. When in doubt eat (or drink) more protein!

How to Set up Your Training Schedule

I'm going to suggest while you take a shot at Bodyweight Training and ignore other training methods, you also ignore any of the ideas on how to schedule your work outs you picked up from mainstream body building and fitness sources.

Try this instead...
"A" Days. Full body Bodyweight Training andchoice of cardio.

1. Warm up and stretching.
2. Pushups. 5 sets.
3. Choice of Dips. 3 sets.
4. Pull Ups. 5 sets.
5. Back Bridges. 3 sets.
6. Bodyweight Squats. 5 sets.
7. Bodyweight Lunges. 3 sets.
8. Leg Raises. 5 sets.
9. Choice of Ab exercise. 3 sets.

Choice of Ab exercise. 3 sets.

"B" Days. Rest - light stretching possibly cardio depending on level of fatigue and need to cut body fat.

Now this is hardly the only choice of how you can set up your Bodyweight Training sessions - you can choose to do your split according to body parts or by some other criteria, but this simple schedule sky rockets metabolism and conditioning levels in everyone I've ever seen use it.

Think outside the box and give it a shot before you try something else. I think you will be seriously glad you did!

For more information about products that can support you on your Journey to Weight loss, & Amazing health visit:

SakuraNutraceuticals.com

Conclusion
The Mind as A Muscle
(Positive Thinking and Goal Setting)

Before we end this Guide, I'm going to reveal what may be the biggest secret of them all when it comes to developing the body of your dreams. It's not exclusive to Bodyweight Training, though it does apply to our beloved form of fitness as much or more so than any of the other many methods.

The secret?

That no matter what you are doing, how hard you are training and how well you are eating and supplementing - if your Mind is not working with you rather than against you, you will never be living up to your fitness potential.

Your Mind is a muscle - the most important muscle of them all in fact when it comes to getting fit!

How can we get our Mind working with us rather than against us while Bodyweight Training? Read on and findout...

The Power of Positive Thinking

Now I'm not trying to go all New Age on you, but facts are facts - when you think positively you are much morelikely to accomplish or surpass your physical goals than when you are drenched in negativity. This is why professional athletes engage in rabid levels of positive self-talk before an event and some even use sports hypnosis to implant positive thoughts in their minds to give them every edge possible.

You've never heard of anyone engaging in negative self-talk before a big Olympic event, have you? Of course not.

How can we take advantage of this in our training? The simplest way is to first try to block out negative thoughts as best we can whenever they pop in our heads.

By following these with a simple affirmation like "Every day am getting stronger, faster, healthier, more attractive and smarter" we really set the foundation for success. Saying the affirmation in a mirror first thing in the morning a few times in front of the mirror as well as before going to sleep at night will pay off huge dividendstoo!

At first you may feel a bit silly when you use your affirmations. I know I did. Once you see how well they work, however, I guarantee you will join me in respecting their power!

Goal Setting and Bodyweight Training

When you set clear and achievable fitness goals (preferably writing them down) you are programming your subconscious mind to join in the fight to get you fit.While Bodyweight Training invest in an inexpensive notebook to use as a journal and be sure to write down weekly, monthly and quarterly training goals.

Are you doing 20 pushups in a set now, but would like tobe up to 35 in a set by the end of the month? Write it down! Is your goal to lose twenty pounds of fat in the nextninety days? Write it down!

As long as these goals are realistic and achievable youwill find yourself achieving many more of them before you began to goal set. It's the way mind works and weshould use it to our advantage whenever possible.

There two simple tactics can get your Mind on board asthe most important muscle of them all. Expect tremendous results!

For the Elite Trainer Advanced Bodyweight Exercises

Welcome to our bonus chapter! Are you ready to try some more advanced Bodyweight Training exercises?These are great for after you establish a strength andfitness foundation and are ready to take things to thenext level.

The idea Bodyweight Training is just for fitness newbies and the inexperienced is so far from true it's laughable. If anyone ever tells you that, challenge them to get their butt off the leg press and have a battle of Burpees. Or to leave the Lat Pulldown alone and try to do a Muscle Up. Should they accept prepare to have a huge laugh at theirexpense!

Incorporate these Advanced Bodyweight Training Exercises into your routine and the world better beware!

The Burpee. The Burpee is a favorite total body

Conditioning exercise as well as cardio builder. Beloved by American and British Special Forces as well as maximum security prisoners (!!!) worldwide. When you can do 500 in a row you are officially approaching superhuman.

1. Stand up straight feet shoulder width apart.
2. Drop into a squat.
3. Kick feet back into a push up position.
4. Lower into push up.

5. Push back up.
6. Kick feet into bottom squat position, explode upward into a jump extending arms overhead.
7. Repeat.

The Hindu Pushup. Also called the Dand this is an exercise that built explosive power in Indian wrestlers fora thousand years. It's now used by mixed martial artists who are addicted to the total body workout it provides.

One of my favorites

1. Feet on the floor hand in pushup position form a "V" with body. This resembles Downward Facing Dog if youare familiar with yoga.
2. Lower yourself down elbows tucked in as if you were ducking under a rope.
3. Immediately curl up your spine as if you were comingup on other side of rope.
4. Return to start position.
5. Hindu pushups are similar to dive bomber pushups which you may have seen at one time or another.

I saved the toughest for last...

The Muscle Up Pullup. Make no mistake when you start pounding out Muscle Ups you are officially a Bodyweight Training master. It takes many fit trainers YEARS to get their first full Muscle Up. If you apply yourself and hit your Pull ups and Dips without fail it won't take you nearly as long, when you are ready here's how they are done:

1. Do a normal pull up, but end as high as possible. Ideally the bar should be touching your waste.
2. Kick (or "kip" to use a CrossFit term) your legs to

give you added momentum if necessary. However, you make itthe goal is to get your body on top of the bar!

3. Immediately do a press up as if you were on dip bars.Lock out your elbows for a second and look at your amazed admirers.
4. Dip down and up again.
5. Return to bottom pull up position.
6. Repeat. If you can!
7. Put video on YouTube. You are now a Bodyweight Training Jedi!

There's plenty more where these come from, but after the basics in our Guide and these extras to look forward to I think you will be busy for quite some time.

Nothing feels better than being able to master your own body and I wanted to say thanks for letting me be your coach for the process.

For more information about products that can support you on your Journey to Weight loss, & Amazing health visit:

SakuraNutraceuticals.com

Bonus Content

How to Overcome Emotional Eating

Eating is a part of life. Your body gets its nutrients from food. Sometimes we can go overboard with our eating habits and it can result in gaining weight. One issue with food is emotional eating.

The problem of emotional eating may end with the scale but it begins in the mind. Stress takes its toll on your life. When your defenses are compromised your health takes a hit and so do your emotions.

Everyone has good days and bad days. How we deal with the bad ones brings emotional eating into play. You look for comfort for your hurts. People who turn to food for comfort find a coping mechanism that won't judge them, hurt them or tell them "no." To complicate the issue, eating pleasurable foods can stimulate the release of endorphins just like exercise. So, after you eat, you feel better.

Emotional eaters use food to relieve stress. They hide behind the food instead of seeking solutions to the problems. This is not uncommon when the stressor is something horrible such as physical abuse or a death.

But, how do you know you are using food in this way? The first sign is obvious. You will gain weight if you eat too much.

In light of the weight gain, examine other areas of your life:

- Have you been under stress lately at work or at home?
- Has anything traumatic happened in the last year?
- Are you dealing with a problem but haven't found a solution?

Answering "yes" to any of these questions could mean that you are an emotional eater. You eat but you are not necessarily hungry at the time. The foods that you choose are what we term "comfort foods":

- High fat foods like French fries, fried foods
- High carb foods like macaroni and cheese, mashed potatoes
- Sugary foods like ice cream, donuts, cookies, cake

There is help for emotional eaters. The first step is recognizing that you have a problem. You'll experience feelings of helplessness and guilt. The guilt is over potentially ruining your health and the helplessness lies in the fact that you don't see a way out.

Secondly, seek counseling. There are many types of counselors out there that can meet your need. Emotional eating has nothing to do with dieting or changing your eating habits but gaining control over your emotions.

A counselor might suggest things like visualization, practicing problem solving skills, relaxation techniques and family support. Visualization helps you to see your problems in a realistic way and not blown out of proportion. You will also learn to see food as nutrition for the body and not an emotional crutch.

Thirdly, your family can learn your triggers for stress and be on the lookout for changes in your eating habits. They can help you be aware of the foods you are eating, assist you in making healthy food choices and exercise along with you. Proper diet and exercise increase immunity, blood flow and positive thinking.

Yoga enhances the mind/body connection so you don't eat when you aren't hungry. Finding new ways to solve your problems and deal with stress will push food out of the equation. You'll feel good about finding solutions which will replace the dependence on food.

The Power of Antioxidants for Staying Young

Everyone wants to grow old gracefully. Some go under the knife to get that youthful look while others opt for a more natural way to maintain that healthful glow. The way to make peace with age can be found in the types of foods that we eat and the miracle ingredient they contain.

This hidden "miracle" is called antioxidants. They have graced the pages of magazines, medical journals and every product from hand cream to supplement pills. But what are antioxidants and what can they do to keep you looking your best?

Antioxidants are substances that fight the aging process that goes on in your body. They are not produced by the body so to get the benefit of these power-packed substances you must ingest them. A variety of foods contain antioxidants.

Let's go back to the beginning. The body continually replenishes its cells. Through a process called cellular metabolism, the body produces energy, more cells and repairs any damage. One by-product of cellular metabolism is unstable molecules called free radicals.

Free radicals are molecules that damage your body. They are unstable because they are missing an electron. To get another one and become stable, free radicals will steal electrons from cells. That theft damages the cells in a variety of ways.

The results are visible and invisible changes to our bodies. The development of diseases like cancer, diabetes, arthritis and neurological deficiencies may begin to affect you as you age. Also, thinner skin wrinkles and brittle bones are a problem. Free radicals enter our body from outside sources as well: cigarette smoke, radiation and the sun's UV rays. The more free radicals we encounter, the greater the damage that can be done.

Antioxidants have been shown to be of great help in the free radical problem. Antioxidant substances combine with free radicals and neutralize them. Once they are neutralized, they can no longer do any damage. Scientists don't have any idea of a recommended daily dose of antioxidants to correct free radical damage and the diseases that come with age, but they do know that eating foods rich in antioxidants makes a huge difference in how we live.

Where do you find antioxidants? They are all around us. Look no further than your local farmer's market or produce aisle in the grocery store. Fruits and vegetables contain the principal sources of antioxidants.

Examples of antioxidants include:

- Vitamin C
- Vitamin A
- Vitamin E
- Lutein
- Lycopene
- Beta-carotene

Certain minerals like zinc and selenium also function in the body. They are not antioxidants but they boost the immune system to fight against free radical damage.

Antioxidants are also found in nuts, legumes, cold water fish, seafood and red meat. So, eating a varied diet of fruits, vegetables and the foods just named will increase the amount of antioxidants in your system and help reduce the incidence of disease. Eating fruits and vegetables in their natural form instead of juices brings the benefit of other nutrients found in the foods. Juices also contain a lot of sugar that is not needed by your body.

Food does more than stave off hunger. Natural substances found there can cause us to live longer and stay free of disease as we age.

Top Ten Power Packed Foods

What is the secret to a long and healthy life? It is in the food that we eat. As you well know, all foods are not created equal. Choosing and eating the right foods may help increase your life expectancy as well as the quality of your life.

Here are ten of the top power packed foods designed to give you energy, vitality and all-around good health!

1. Beans – If they give you gas, take precautions before you eat them. Soaking them first can help. Beans of all kinds (kidney, navy, lentils, chickpeas, Northern) are high in protein. This is plant protein so it contains very little fat, carbs and calories. If fiber is a problem in your diet, eating a healthy portion of beans each day can keep your digestive system healthy.
2. Oatmeal – Oatmeal is coming into popularity as a food that lowers blood cholesterol. You can make it yourself with rolled oats or eat the instant kind if you are in a hurry. Oatmeal is a filling grain that also provides much needed fiber to keep hunger at bay and your blood sugar constant.

3. Fruits – Fruits are filled with antioxidants such as Vitamin C and A. Antioxidants fight free radical damage in the body and reduce the risk of cancer. Berries such as blueberries and grapes have the highest amount of antioxidants. But choose an array of fruits in a wide variety of colors for maximum health. The antioxidants in fruit boost the immune system to fight the effects of aging in the body.

4. Allium foods – This class of foods includes garlic, onions, leeks and shallots. Garlic is known for lowering cholesterol. Allium vegetables help guard the body against the risk of cancer and many other ailments. They also help lower blood pressure and prevent blood clots. Eating these power packed vegetables in their natural state especially garlic increases their health benefits.

5. Salmon – Eating foods rich in omega-3 fatty acids reduces the risk of heart disease and other conditions like atherosclerosis. Wild salmon is a fatty fish but it contains good fats that has been proven to improve health in children and adults. Salmon is rich in

protein which is of great use after an exercise session to build muscle tissue.

6. Flax seed – Like salmon it contains omega-3 fatty acids. These seeds also contain omega-6 and omega-9 fatty acids. You get a lot of power to fight high cholesterol, heart disease and diabetes with this seed. Ground flax seed can be added to fruit smoothies, sprinkled in yogurt, eaten with cereal or added to pancake mix to name a few.

7. Peppers – Peppers are colorful. They contain antioxidants like beta-carotene and Vitamin C. Peppers range from mild and sweet to so hot you'll be calling the fire department. All peppers contain a substance called capsaicin. Capsaicin has the properties of an anti-inflammatory, a pain reliever, lowers cancer risk and heart disease. They are good in salads, salsa and all sorts of dishes.

8. Nuts and seeds – Nuts are high in fat but those fats are the good kind. Peanuts, almonds, Brazil nuts, walnuts and pistachios are all providers of good fats and protein. Crush them into a fine powder and use as a coating instead of higher carb bread crumbs. Nuts help to lower cholesterol. Eat them right out of the shell with no additives.

9. Açai – This berry has been in the news lately. It is rich in antioxidants and increases energy. You can get more done and look better while doing it. You can get Acai juice and supplements in your health food store.

10. Yogurt – The fat free variety is good for you. Yogurt contains calcium, Vitamin B, and protein. If you don't drink milk, yogurt is an alternative to get your

calcium in to build strong bones and teeth. Live yogurt also contains friendly bacteria to help promote a healthy digestive system.

Building a better healthier body begins with what you eat. Try these super foods to get started on the right foot.

Five Easy Toning Exercises you can Do Anywhere

Exercise is an important part of our lives. Staying in shape is one way to increase your life expectancy. Weight bearing exercises are important also for increasing muscle mass and bone density as you age.

Most of us have learned what to do when it comes to exercising. The problem is where and when to get the job done. With a busy lifestyle, making time for exercise is a challenge.

Weight bearing exercises aren't just for bodybuilders. As you age, especially once you hit the age of forty, you begin to lose muscle mass. For women especially, bone loss becomes a problem. When the body is in need of calcium it can rob it from your bones. Building muscle not only increases their mass but your strength.

Here are five easy toning exercises that can be done anywhere and whenever you have time. At home, at the office, or on vacation, you can do these easy yet extremely effective exercises.

1. The Bridge Butt Lift – Sounds like a plastic surgery technique but it is an easy way to tone your buttocks. Lay down with feet flat on the floor, legs

shoulder width apart. Place your hands, palm side down, on either side of your body. Pushing with your feet, squeeze your gluteal muscles and lift your butt off the floor. Hold the position for a count of five to ten and release down to the floor.

2. Squats – Squats work the butt, the hamstring muscles and the quadriceps. If you aren't sure of proper form, you can use a chair. Stand with feet shoulder width apart and feet firmly planted. Push your butt back as if you were preparing to sit in a chair. Keep your abs tight and your upper body straight. Once you reach chair level stop and hold the position for a count of two to five and release. At the lowest point, place all of your weight on your heels for balance and maximum toning.

3. Reverse Lunges – Lunges work the quadriceps muscles. They can be hard for people with knee problems. A reverse lunge still tones the right muscle groups but with less pressure on the knee. Stand with feet together and arms at your sides. Take one leg and move it backwards until you are in lunge position: front leg bent at a 90-degree angle and back leg extended until you are on the ball of your foot. From this position lower yourself down until the back knee almost touches the floor. Hold for a count of two and return to starting position.

4. Pushups – This is a classic toning exercise that works all areas of the arms plus the chest muscles. If you aren't comfortable or strong enough to perform a pushup on your toes, lower your body to your knees. Be sure your arms are tucked into the body and your back straight as you lower and lift your body.

5. Crunches – Abdominal muscles can be worked every day to build strength and muscle tone. Lying on the floor in sit up position, lace your fingers behind your head. Squeezing your abdominal muscles, lift your upper body until your lower back is about to come off the floor. Hold for two to five counts and return to starting position.

These five exercise moves can be done whenever you have time. The best thing about exercise is that its effects are cumulative. Even five or ten minutes at a time will work to your advantage.

The Benefits of Exercise Go Beyond Weight Loss

Whether you want to lose a few or a hundred pounds, it's crucial that you understand that the benefits of exercise go way beyond weight loss and cosmetic enhancement. Some benefits of exercise pertain to your health in particular.

Exercising often (3-4 times a week, an hour and a half at least each day) has been found by experts to greatly reduce the risk of several diseases and health conditions. Some diseases that exercise will help you prevent are heart disease, stroke, and Peripheral Vascular Disease.

High blood pressure and high cholesterol are both health conditions that could be avoided by regular exercise. Diabetes that's non-insulin-dependent can be controlled by eliminating most body fat and increasing your daily physical activity.

Over 40% of American people alone are considered medically obese.

This is caused by a lack of activity in your everyday life and the increase in fast food in our diets. By building muscle mass rather than fat, it will help your metabolism increase, which makes burning calories easy.

Most patients that come into a doctor's office complaining of back pain are overweight. Doing exercises that improve your flexibility; such as yoga, Pilates, and tai chi, for example will be able to help reduce back pain.

The benefits of exercise clearly go beyond weight loss. It's more than just making your body look great - it also makes your life-span increasingly longer so that you can enjoy your loved ones and all that life has to offer.

What's the Difference Between Aerobic Exercise and Anaerobic Exercise?

Find yourself in limbo every time your trainer tells you to make sure you do anaerobic exercise this weekend? You aren't the only one confused by the different types. There are many differences between aerobic exercise and anaerobic exercise.

The scientific definition of aerobic is "with oxygen," and anaerobic means without oxygen. Don't take these definitions literally and stop holding your breath! When doing an anaerobic exercise, your body must rely on energy-creating repetitions of exercise that don't need extreme quantities of oxygen. This makes anaerobic exercise very brief and very fast.

Aerobic exercise tones muscles and burns fat. Aerobic exercise gives you a stronger heart, which reduces the risk of cardiovascular disease. It makes your legs and calves more toned, which will make you look great in your little black dress. It also makes that size 6 polka-dot bikini you've been trying to squeeze into obtainable.

Anaerobic exercise makes your bones stronger. Anaerobic exercise also increases your speed and power, as well as giving you increased muscle mass and strength (for all your body builders out there).

It's crucial that you know the difference between aerobic exercise and anaerobic exercise. This way, when your trainer asks what aerobic exercise workouts you did over the weekend, you can tell him – but more important, you'll know that you're giving your body exactly what it needs to achieve optimal health!

Examples of aerobic exercise are running, skiing, rowing, swimming, or even doing an exercise video. Some great examples of anaerobic exercise are tennis, lifting weights, jumping (jumping jacks count), and/or sprinting.

Five Fun Exercises You Can Do Outdoors

Want to know five fun exercises you can do outdoors? When you're outdoors, it makes it more fun to exercise since you can focus your mind on other things instead of how much your legs burn.

Swimming is one of the top five fun exercises you can do outdoors. Swimming works many aspects of your body: your lungs, legs, and arm muscles - not to mention it greatly strengthens the most important body part - your heart.

Swimming allows you to get a great workout without having your body weigh you down with every move you make.

Hiking is also one of many fun exercises you do outdoors. There are many benefits of hiking - not just helping you control your body weight - but also improving your mental health as well. Pack a small, healthy lunch and set up a picnic once you reach a good resting spot.

Rock Climbing is another one of the top five fun exercises you can do outdoors. While you can do rock climbing inside, it's always better to get some fresh air. Rock climbing works mostly your arms and legs, but it also helps your lungs learn how to breathe better.

Biking is fun because you can do it basically anywhere, anytime! You can enjoy the scenery by yourself or you can bring a friend along. Just make sure you always wear your helmet for extra safety precautions while you get your workout in.

Obstacle courses are a great form of fun exercises. They work almost all aspects of your body and with each turn on the course, you can try to be faster. This will help you build endurance. These activities that you do outdoors will replace your fitness boredom with some healthy fun exercise activity!

How to Make Exercise Less Boring

Tired of the same old 12 reps, 10 squats, and 20 minutes on the treadmill? There *is* a way to make exercise less boring! If you're sick of walking on a flat surface on your treadmill, there are many ways to liven up that work out.

Putting on an hour-long TV show that you have to get involved in is a great way to make your mind wander. While watching your show, set your pace at a very light jog. When a commercial comes on, pick up your pace then slow back down when the show returns.

Another way to make exercise less boring is to add other things to make it exciting. Add people or music. Set your iPod to shuffle and get moving. Create various exercise playlists and then don't stop until the music does.

Adding people to your workout is another way to make exercise less boring. Generally, people have five times more chance of taking the initiative to even *go* to the gym when they're with a friend - and are ten times more likely to *continue* going to the gym when they have a partner to help motivate them.

Rewarding yourself when you do a good job at the gym is a key element of making exercise less boring. Don't get too excited - this doesn't mean you can have a whole box of Twinkies. This means that after a long and strenuous workout, you can treat yourself to a massage at a spa or a new outfit to suit that trimmer, healthier figure you're now sporting.

If You Can Buy, One Piece of Exercise Equipment, Get This!

If you're on a budget but need just one piece of exercise equipment you can use day after day - get a treadmill. Treadmills are the best pieces of exercise equipment out there because everyone can use them to the degree that suits your cardiovascular needs. Believe it or not, treadmills are multi-use machines.

Treadmills can be used rain or shine – so no more weather excuses. You can take a long walk, quick run, or medium-length jog and be able to just jump off whenever you please instead of having to turn around and go back to where you came from.

This piece of exercise equipment is also helpful because it makes your heart stronger. When you run on the treadmill, your heart pumps out blood faster and faster - the more pumps, the stronger it gets. It's been said that fitness is the best way to get healthy, that exercise will out-perform medicine in many cases.

A treadmill is a great piece of exercise equipment because it burns fat fast. According to experts across the country, the treadmill burns the most calories out of all other exercise equipment - beating out thing such as rowing machines, stair machines, and even the elliptical depending on how you use it.

Many may argue that these pieces of exercise equipment, while effective, may not be as good for you as a walk outdoors because they don't give you the ups and downs of a normal road, but they're mistaken.

Almost all treadmills that are sold now have resistance training (uphill, downhill slants) and have different workout options such as fat burner, marathon training, and more that will create a variety in your walking instead of just walking on a flat surface.

Exercise Toys for the Home Gym

Are you lucky enough to be able to have your own home gym but are unsure of what exactly to put into it? Or do you have enough space to work out in, but aren't sure what exercise equipment will fit into your living space? Here are some exercise toys that will finally make your home gym complete.

If you have a home gym with a cable pulley, then there are many great exercise toys to add onto that. One of them is a rope attachment. This makes triceps press downs easier to perform. This is also great to replace a lat bar that is generally used for triceps press downs.

Other great exercise toys for the home gym are fun things such as yoga or exercise balls. These help many aspects of your body, most important the core strength you build. These balls can be used in combination with DVDs (that may or may not come with it) or they could also be used to create your own workout regimens.

Yoga mats also make nice exercise toys for your home gym. They come in many colors and sizes - you can pick them according to your taste and what you will be using them for.

An E-Z Bar is another great addition to your home gym. In many fitness and exercise stores, these can be found for under $40. The E-Z Bar allows you to enhance your workout as well as create a new one. Curls can be interchanged with E-Z Bar Curls in order to work the biceps from a different angle.

Other great additions to a home gym include steps, various dumbbell sets, and stretch ropes. Just have to find the ones that are right for you.

For more information about products that can support you on your Journey to Weight loss, & Amazing health visit:

SakuraNutraceuticals.com

Made in the USA
Monee, IL
04 November 2026

67387552R00085